CCSVI as the Cause
of Multiple Sclerosis

T0130856

McFarland Health Topics Series

CCSVI as the Cause of Multiple Sclerosis

The Science Behind the Controversial Theory

MARIE A. RHODES

Foreword by E. Mark Haacke

MCFARLAND HEALTH TOPICS SERIES
Elaine A. Moore, *Series Editor*

McFarland & Company, Inc., Publishers
Jefferson, North Carolina, and London

LIBRARY OF CONGRESS CATALOGUING-IN-PUBLICATION DATA

Rhodes, Marie A., 1960–
    CCSVI as the cause of multiple sclerosis : the science
behind the controversial theory / Marie A. Rhodes ;
foreword by E. Mark Haacke.
       p.   cm. — (McFarland Health Topics)
    [Elaine A. Moore, series editor]
    Includes bibliographical references and index.

    ISBN 978-0-7864-6038-0
    softcover : 50# alkaline paper ∞

    1. Multiple Sclerosis — etiology.   2. Cerebral Veins —
physiopathology.   3. Multiple Sclerosis — therapy.
4. Spinal Cord — blood supply.   5. Venous Insufficency —
complications.   I. Title.
RC377.R47   2011
616.8'34 — dc22   2011008713

BRITISH LIBRARY CATALOGUING DATA ARE AVAILABLE

Front cover image © 2011 Shutterstock

Manufactured in the United States of America

McFarland & Company, Inc., Publishers
  Box 611, Jefferson, North Carolina 28640
  www.mcfarlandpub.com

Table of Contents

Acknowledgments

The first and most important person I would like to thank is Paolo Zamboni, MD, of Ferrara, Italy, whose incredible discovery makes this book possible. This gentle man, who suffers from a neurodegenerative disease of his own, truly understands what it's like to live with a physical challenge. He has devoted his time to educating other medical professionals about his findings while he simultaneously participates in additional research to find further answers about how CCSVI contributes to multiple sclerosis. Dr. Zamboni very kindly reviewed the manuscript of this book before publication and was available to me for questions as I wrote. My gratitude to him is heartfelt.

Next I would like to thank E. Mark Haacke, PhD, the world-renowned physicist and pioneer in MR imaging. This award-winning researcher became interested in the CCSVI model when he learned of Dr. Zamboni's work because his extensive research involving imaging iron in the brains of MS patients, begun in 1997, is potentially supportive of the new model. Dr. Haacke's dedication to evaluating CCSVI has included establishing an innovative worldwide registry to record data gathered in a very specific imaging protocol which evaluates blood flow before and after angioplasty treatment for CCSVI. Dr. Haacke made himself available to me and not only reviewed an early draft along and offered recommendations for making the book better, but also kindly performed a complete review of the final manuscript. I am very grateful for the generous gift of Dr. Haacke's time and thoughtful consideration of my work.

The next person I would like to thank is Marian Simka, MD, a vascular specialist and researcher in Poland. He was one of the first physicians to undertake treatment for CCSVI and his research in this field has helped answer important questions about this new paradigm. When I contacted him regarding some of his research he thoughtfully offered to review my work. His kind encouragement and assurance that a book that reviews the research related to CCSVI would be a valuable contribution gave me the heart to press on. I am very appreciative of Dr. Simka's mentorship.

I would also like to thank Michael Dake, MD, who not only generously reviewed portions of this book but who also performed my own angioplasty for CCSVI in his observational study of the new model. I do not believe I could have undertaken this monumental task before that procedure; my improved energy has changed my life for the better. I will be forever grateful to this compassionate physician, and he holds a special place in my heart for his willingness to treat me.

Several other physicians have reviewed portions of the book. I would like to thank Jack Burks, MD, for his review and kind words about the chapter on immunology. I would also like to thank David Hubbard, MD, for his generous review and critique of chapters one and six and Gianfranco Campalani, MD, for encouragement after reviewing an early draft.

These medical professionals provided me with critical support and clarification of their research to make sure that my words accurately reflected their intention.

I have also had kind and generous support from professionals in the publishing industry. I would like to thank my editor Elaine A. Moore who generously took me under her wing and supported me not only by editing my work, but also by sending me books and magazines from her personal library to help me write more clearly. She also referred me to Marv Miller, a medical illustrator she had worked with on previous projects. His generous offer to read the book then design illustrations for those places where readers could use visual aid was invaluable to the final version of this book. I'm very grateful to both of these people.

In addition to this professional support, many MS patients kindly reviewed the manuscript. The first MS patient that I'd like to thank is my friend Samantha Wilkinson, who wrote a book with Elaine Moore for McFarland titled *The Promise of Low Dose Naltrexone Therapy*. When she was asked to write another book about MS, she suggested McFarland might like to contact me. The result was a contract to write this book. Sam generously reviewed multiple drafts and was always ready with a kind word. Many times when I wondered what I was doing, Sam reassured me that patients would love this book, and she suggested the plain language summaries at the end of each chapter as a way to help make the dense science more understandable. I will always be grateful to Sam; without her help this book could never have happened.

The other patients I would like to thank are all of the people who contributed their stories to chapter 7. Jeff, Sharon, Carrie, Mark, Melissa, Lew, Gianfranco, Devin and Danielle generously allowed readers to take a peek into their personal lives by sharing their stories in this book. In addition to offering their stories, Sharon, Mark, Lew and Danielle read the complete manuscript and gave me feedback about how patients might read this book. The ideas that they shared with me helped make the book more readable to nonmedical people.

Finally, I would like to thank the members of my family who supported me throughout this process. First, my daughter reviewed the book and contributed insightful comments and also handled some of the typing that was difficult for me because of my disability. My sister read the entire manuscript and shared very helpful suggestions for smoothing out the chapters. My son developed a sixth sense about when I needed food or fluid and was good about bringing those things to me.

And last but most important I would like to thank the person who truly made it all possible — my husband Bill Rhodes. This exceptional man supported me and took care of our life so that I could be free to work on this project. He also took care of numerous things I could not do for myself and he never said to me that I was too disabled to do a project like this; he simply made it possible. I am truly blessed to know such a wonderful person and will be forever grateful that he sees something in me beyond my disability.

I am truly grateful to have had the generous support of so many kind people. My heartfelt thanks goes to each and every person; thank you.

Foreword by
E. Mark Haacke

Breakthroughs in research sometimes happen very fast by insightful new concepts, such as the discovery of insulin by Banting and Macleod in 1922 (for which they won the 1923 Nobel Prize in Physiology and Medicine). Within a very short time it became clear that the discovery of insulin would have an important clinical impact for patients. Yet the recognition of such breakthroughs does not always come so easy, as in the example of the bacteria that causes ulcers as promoted by Warren and Marshall (for which they won the 2005 Nobel Prize in Physiology). Sometimes it is necessary to overcome such strong beliefs that it takes years and even decades to demonstrate an obvious truth. Sometimes it is nothing more than taking the right perspective to apply some extra knowledge that allows one to jump into a heliocentric universe from the archaic belief of a geocentric system.

So it may be with the role of the vasculature in the human brain and the role of the cardiovasculature in affecting the human brain. Thus believed Tracey J. Putnam in 1935 and so believed Paolo Zamboni, MD, in 2009, both extolling the role of venous hypertension in multiple sclerosis (MS). Interestingly, our understanding of the role of the vasculature, its fluid dynamics and its hemodynamics, is so limited that there is no single textbook devoted to a comprehensive understanding of its role in brain function. We are still at the cutting edge of such research, but today, unlike Putnam's day, we have the tools to investigate the vasculature *in vivo* in both healthy and vascularly impaired individuals.

With modern imaging tools such as ultrasound, magnetic resonance imaging (MRI) and computed tomography, we can non-invasively image the human body, including the entire cardiovascular system, both anatomically and functionally. Using these tools as a means to study the major veins in the brain today has led to a large cohort of physicians worldwide treating these major chronic cerebrospinal venous insufficiency (CCSVI) venous abnormal-

1

ities with percutaneous transluminal angioplasty. Currently there are a number of ongoing studies around the world set in motion to try and validate the findings of Professor Zamboni and quantify the frequency of stenoses, the flow abnormalities in both multiple sclerosis patients and in normal volunteers, and the recovery of those patients treated with angioplasty.

This book is an overview of the history of the role of veins in multiple sclerosis, the current status of some of the research related to CCSVI, the politics that have ensconced it during the last year, patient testimonials, and current directions in imaging and treatment. It will be a valuable resource for medical professionals and patients seeking information to understand the new paradigm.

Time will tell how important the vascular system is in MS and how these endovascular treatments have helped MS patients. No doubt the vascular system is so complicated that there will be much to learn in both understanding and treating CCSVI. This thrust will have direct implications not only for understanding MS better, for treating MS patients, and for monitoring MS patients, but also for the importance of the vascular system to neurodegenerative disease in general. It won't be long before we will be looking forward to the second edition of this book once the first episodes in this story have unfolded.

E. Mark Haacke is the author of MRI: Physical Principals and Sequence Design; *editor of the first text in MR angiography with Dr. James Potchen; and editor of* Current Protocols in MRI. *Director of the MRI Institute for Biomedical Research, and director of the MR research facility at Wayne State University, he is a professor at Wayne State, Loma Linda University, Case Western Reserve, and McMaster University.*

Preface — How to Use This Book

For Nonmedical Readers

This book is written for people interested in CCSVI whether they have a medical background or not. I have included several features to make this information easy to understand for nonmedical readers; every chapter has a plain-language summary at the end and I also include a glossary and index. Some readers may prefer to start with the plain-language summary, then read the chapter. The book is best read from front to back.

The last three chapters of this book provide information directly applicable to people who are considering consulting a vascular physician for evaluation and potential treatment. These chapters provide the reader with a background to participate in discussions about that possibility with his or her doctor. The information included leans toward risks and information readers should understand to be equal partners in such discussions, while the patient stories provide a hopeful look at the possibilities.

The appendix provides a guide, written by Dr. Haacke himself, that allows people in an institutional review board (IRB) trial using the Haacke imaging protocol to understand their patient report. Chapter 8 also includes information readers could give to intrigued physicians so they can be part of this trial creating a local resource.

For Medical Professionals

The studies offered by the research team led by Dr. Zamboni have challenged the mainstream view of MS. In this book I review medical literature related to MS from the venous perspective to provide a broad understanding of the venous model.

While the first chapter documents the political environment around this new model, subsequent chapters are focused on a review of the evidence base.

3

Some medical professionals might assume on first glance that chapters 2 and 3 covering the existing evidence base for MS are old news, but this book offers a broad review of this foundation that constantly brings in the venous perspective. This fresh review of the history and epidemiology of MS challenges the medical professional to reevaluate how the current paradigm became predominant and to consider the longstanding evidence that supports the venous model.

I read and referenced well over 200 peer-reviewed papers to support the statements in this book and my hope is that it will spark the interest of other medical professionals to further evaluate Dr. Zamboni's premise. With this in mind I also included the PubMed identification numbers in the bibliography.

Introduction

The lives of MS patients may soon change dramatically based on a new medical discovery. According to new research, it appears that occlusions in the veins contribute to the disease process and pathology in MS. This newly described anomaly, which has been demonstrated in the veins of individuals with MS, is called chronic cerebrospinal venous insufficiency, or CCSVI. This book offers a comprehensive look at this new research.

The Italian vascular expert and researcher Paolo Zamboni, MD, first recognized the significance of this finding and then advanced this medical discovery. As a professor of vascular surgery and director of the Vascular Center at the University of Ferrara, Italy, as well as an internationally-recognized vascular researcher, this physician is well qualified to consider multiple sclerosis from a vascular perspective.

Dr. Zamboni also has a personal reason for wanting to fully understand this disease and find efficacious treatment; his own wife has multiple sclerosis.

My own interest in this new theory was inspired by the need for a new way to address my progressive MS; however, as I am a registered nurse (RN), my interest in new ideas always includes a critical evaluation of the associated peer-reviewed medical literature.

With this bias, I undertook the task of a complete review of the new CCSVI model, starting with learning about related research from vascular medicine and working through all of Dr. Zamboni's research, his references, and pertinent related papers. I read hundreds of research papers over the course of a year. What I discovered as I investigated this model sparked my enthusiasm and formed the framework for this book.

Though CCSVI is a radical departure from the traditional view, which holds that MS is purely an autoimmune disease, Dr. Zamboni's extensive years-long research offers a compelling case which suggests that a more accurate way of thinking about MS therapy should include evaluation and treatment of vascular anomalies as part of comprehensive MS patient care.

Treatment of venous malformations such as those Dr. Zamboni describes is currently available, even though it will be some years before it will be clear exactly how the immune system and these newly revealed venous changes interact to cause MS. As a result of this lack of clarity, neurologists consider such treatment highly controversial even though vascular physicians consider angioplasty for similar problems routinely.

The controversy finds its roots in the fact that neurologists deem current treatment of multiple sclerosis highly scientific and evidence-based even though such treatment does not cure MS. This book reviews this evidence base with a critical eye, highlighting weaknesses in the traditional model and placing special emphasis on existing research that supports the idea that the new venous model is an important advancement in complete understanding of this disease.

In reality, there has always been evidence of a venous component to multiple sclerosis even though this extensive evidence had been largely ignored prior to this time. This fact lends added credence to the new research done in Italy.

Later chapters undertake in-depth review and discussion of the new research offered by the Italian research team headed by Dr. Zamboni. This is also balanced by discussion of weaknesses in the new theory as well as opposing research offered by critics. The result is a big-picture view of how the new venous model may be seen, taking into account the wider MS evidence base.

People evaluating this new research and treatment model will also presumably be interested in learning about treatment of venous problems with angioplasty. With this in mind, I have provided information about angioplasty, including issues that patients should be aware of as part of their consideration. Though vascular physicians such as interventional radiologists consider angioplasty routine, informed patients are more able to participate in meaningful discussion with these professionals.

The last part of the book is highlighted by stories of patients who have been treated and can speak of their experience more than a year after treatment, including changes in their lives as a result of this new approach. My own story is included as I was treated early in 2009.

Finally, this book includes unique resources. These resources include information readers can take to local vascular doctors so that those who are interested can participate in a trial and treat people with MS for CCSVI. There is also a detailed explanation of how to read the patient report if readers should be in a trial or see a physician using the Haacke imaging protocol, as well as information on ways to get involved with the activist patient community that is working to demand immediate, open-minded and thorough evaluation of this new idea should readers wish to participate.

One way people with MS and their advocates are making a difference is by supporting those entities established to raise funds for the extensive research that is needed to clarify how exactly CCSVI is involved with the MS process. Many different ways people can get involved in contributing to this effort are outlined in chapter 8, from small and simple to large. Together, MS patients and their advocates are making a difference. I am personally volunteering on the patient board of CCSVI Alliance, a 501(3)(c) charity dedicated to helping raise funds for research of CCSVI.

I am also contributing 10 percent of my proceeds from this book directly to research of CCSVI through CCSVI Alliance.

This book is educational in nature and not to be taken as medical advice. It is intended to empower patients, to provide them with a background on the theory of CCSVI in MS so they may follow the research as it develops, and to help prepare them for discussions with their own trusted medical advisors. The information included in this book is the author's opinion, not the mainstream view, and may not apply to individual situations. Please consult your own medical professional for recommendations suitable to your situation.

1

The Politics of Change

How do you turn a chunk of coal into a diamond? Steady pressure and time.
Since we are all running out of time, we need a lot of steady pressure — posted
on ThisIsMS.com (TIMS)

There are big changes taking place in the multiple sclerosis (MS) community. This disease, which doctors traditionally thought to be purely autoimmune, suddenly appears to have a significant vascular component. Research conducted in Italy by the vascular surgeon Paolo Zamboni, MD, suggests that the veins leading from the brain and spinal cord in MS patients have significant blockages that vascular doctors could repair in a simple outpatient procedure. Some MS patients have had such procedures and highlights of their experiences are shared later in this chapter and in chapter 7.

Patients worldwide have embraced this new avenue of research and potential treatment with activist exuberance while neurologists look on in disbelief, dismayed as patients unexpectedly question their philosophy. The politics of medicine is changing.

"Politics" in this context refers to the ways in which people and institutions relate to each other, the dynamics and flavor of those interactions, the concerns regarding who has power, and the ways in which decisions influence the other players. In medicine there are many stakeholders, ranging from pharmaceutical companies to charitable societies, clinics, physicians of different specialties, research scientists and, of course, MS patients themselves. As research related to the vascular aspect of MS progresses, all of these stakeholders are finding that their traditional positions and the influence they used to wield have shifted.

Prior to the Italian research team's discovery of the vascular defect, which they have labeled chronic cerebrospinal venous insufficiency (CCSVI), MS had been widely accepted as purely autoimmune. As a result, MS care was under the sole command of neurologists, and treatment was based on pharmaceutical approaches that suppress function of the immune system.

Naturally, this new way of looking at MS through a vascular lens has garnered skepticism among neurologists and pharmaceutical companies because they see the new idea as totally unrelated to the theory they had come to accept and that they felt was showing promise. They had come to believe that the autoimmune theory was unassailable.

It is not surprising that the first neurologists to express a public opinion about CCSVI took a purely defensive posture. A reporter interviewed a prominent MS neurologist researcher regarding media coverage of Dr. Zamboni's research and quoted him as follows: "I think there are going to be millions of dollars spent now to follow a hoax" (Blackwell 2010).

This unfortunate comment polarized MS patients interested in CCSVI who felt it revealed a self-serving rejection of the new direction of research rather than the expected excitement about a potential breakthrough. Other neurology researchers cautioned that treatment of occlusions (blockages in the vein) should be halted until neurologists have conducted their own research and concluded that treatment targeting venous occlusion alters the course of multiple sclerosis. As one team of neurologists recommended in an article written in the journal *Neurology*, "At present, invasive and potentially dangerous endovascular procedures as therapy for patients with MS should be discouraged until such studies have been completed, analyzed, and debated in the scientific arena" (Khan et al. 2010).

Such research as these neurologists are recommending would take 5 to 10 years. This unwillingness by some people in the MS field to accept Dr. Zamboni's findings as relevant to patients who may have these occlusions today ignores the fact that healthy circulation has value in its own right. It also neglects the fact that evaluation to check blood flow is currently available from vascular physicians.

Modern research into a vascular connection with the process that results in MS began in 2006 and is still in its early stages. However, researchers worldwide are consistently showing that the majority of people with MS do have blockages or stenoses causing impaired circulation in the veins that lead from the brain and spinal cord, whereas most apparently healthy people do not show evidence of these issues (see chapter 5). Repairing such blockages is a common practice in other parts of the body affected by similar occlusions, using a relatively simple outpatient procedure called angioplasty that restores healthy circulation.

Researchers have not yet completed blinded trials to prove that repairing the blocked veins in CCSVI will make a difference to the disease course in MS. Although the early results from a recent open-label (unblinded) study seem promising, the people treated for CCSVI to date have not generated enough data to establish any scientific conclusion. It will take many studies before researchers can tease out the complex interplay of the immune and venous elements of MS.

Patients have the biggest stake in the debate regarding vascular treatment in MS. Neurologists, vascular specialists, pharmaceutical companies, and the National Multiple Sclerosis Society (NMSS) have a stake in the outcome of this debate as well.

No one can blame the stakeholders for wanting to be involved in answering these questions. It is of vital importance to them, and each group wants to control the discussion according to their own viewpoint. Everyone wants to be heard.

Patients as Stakeholders

On May 5, 2010, a group of Canadians, many in wheelchairs or using other assistive devices, assembled on the street in front of government offices in Queens Park in Toronto, Ontario (Green 2010). This atypical group of protesters held signs demanding that physicians treat them as anyone else with a venous disorder and not as a special class of citizens requiring permission from MS researchers to obtain vascular treatment. Cars passing the area honked, and the protesters waved canes and signs in an exuberant display of empowered people who for a long time had felt powerless and hopeless.

MS patients organized protests such as this via the Internet and synchronized them to occur all over the world on May 5. The patients wanted lawmakers to intervene so that vascular specialists would be free to evaluate and treat vascular occlusions in MS patients without fear of reprisal.

In at least one institution, prominent MS researchers took credit for halting observational research and treatment of CCSVI conducted by an interventional radiologist in their own institution's vascular department. One of the researchers, in describing his role, said, "After sustained and explicit calls to suspend this unproven procedure, we succeeded on December 5" (Samson 2010). The interviewed neurologist believed this was a justified action for the good of MS patients. Clearly, MS patients had other thoughts on this matter.

The protesters asserted that individuals should receive unrestricted assessment and appropriate treatment from vascular specialists based on their own diagnostic tests. They further asserted they should not be required to wait for the neurologists to agree that such testing and treatment is justified. Patients following the development of CCSVI research were particularly incensed that a few neurologists seemed to believe that they were in charge of the entire discussion.

In Canada, patient activism and assertive letter-writing campaigns resulted in the Canadian Parliament inviting vascular specialists to speak on the subject of treatment for CCSVI in MS patients. A prominent Canadian vascular surgeon, Dr. Sandy MacDonald, testified, "This is not a new drug, not a new procedure not a new anything. Angiosplasty has been available since 1984. Hundreds of thousands of procedures have been done. It is not new" (MacDonald 2010).

Angioplasty is the most common medical intervention in the world; over two million procedures are performed each year (Cohen 2003). Dr. Mac-Donald also created a metaphor that patients have now popularized by saying the situation is like having blocked plumbing in a house but the homeowner for some inexplicable reason must ask permission from the electrician before the plumber may fix the pipes.

On June 15, 2010, the Canadian Institute for Health Research announced that it would intervene. In a decision widely applauded by MS patients, they announced the appropriation of funding to investigate the connection between MS and CCSVI, including a resolution of conflicts in the literature. They also proposed an international committee be formed to decide what direction research needs to take next (CTV Winnipeg 2010b).

Patient Dissatisfaction

The controversy surrounding the role of CCSVI in MS pathology and the potential effectiveness of vascular treatment acted as a trigger, evoking the dissatisfaction and feelings of helplessness many patients had been experiencing with the direction of MS patient care. The reasons for the powerful patient activism seen surrounding CCSVI are not entirely rooted in the current debate. Rather, they stem from frustration regarding the effectiveness of pharmaceutical therapies for MS.

People with MS live with an unpredictable disease, and they also live with the effects and consequences of treatment; the side effects of most MS drugs range from affecting quality of life by causing a chronic flu-like reaction to life-threatening consequences such as progressive multifocal leukoencephalopathy (PML), an opportunistic brain infection caused by suppression of the immune system (Berger and Houff 2009). Some patients are required to have additional medical procedures and tests because of what are termed iatrogenic effects, meaning problems caused by doctors or treatment. In addition, many people prescribed MS medications do not feel well on a day-to-day basis. A significant amount of patient distress and dissatisfaction is due to the effects of treatment aimed at altering immune system function and not the disease. The cost of medical intervention is high on many levels.

In spite of this, the arsenal of drugs approved for MS has not been proven to prevent permanent losses of function. A follow-up study on patients who took an interferon drug over 16 years compared these treated people to individuals who had not taken the drug. The researchers found no difference in the percentage of people who had reached progressive disability over those 16 years; in both groups it was roughly 35 percent (Ebers et al. 2010). Another prominent MS researcher comments that although the standard pharmaceutical compounds prescribed for MS usually reduce relapses and inflammatory lesions, sometimes dramatically, no drug has ever been shown to prevent disease progression (Pittock et al. 2006).

Many patients with MS have seen this loss of function occur among their peers at the local NMSS group as people who assumed their disease was stable slip over the invisible line and move into progressive disease and heightened disability. Add to this those peers whose immunosuppressive treatment caused a side effect such as heart disease or leukemia, and it becomes frighteningly clear that MS can hurt people from both sides: the disease itself *and* treatment.

Contrary to this reality of living with MS and the current therapies, glossy ads in the NMSS magazine and in physicians' offices depict smiling people hiking on beautiful mountaintops with the subtitle suggesting that the advertised drug made this possible. These ads are in stark contrast to real MS life for all but the newly diagnosed who are unaware it is common to have mild disease for years after diagnosis, even if untreated (Pittock et al. 2006; see also Confavreux and Vukusic 2006a, 2006b).

When discussion of CCSVI sprang to life among the online MS community forum members, this simmering dissatisfaction with the current disease model evolved into a mutiny, particularly when the initial comments from the neurology community seemed derisive of Dr. Zamboni's work (Khan et al. 2010; Carlson 2010; Blackwell 2010).

In a *New York Times* article about the CCSVI breakthrough, an NMSS official provided a perfect example of the disconnect between people guiding the direction of MS research and the views of patients: "Joyce Nelson, the president of the Multiple Sclerosis Society in the United States, said, 'I wasn't aware how thin the veneer was and how close to the surface the frustration was'" (Grady 2010).

In some patients' views, the frustrating reality is that the society that is supposed to advocate for them seems out of touch.

Patient Advocacy and the National Multiple Sclerosis Society (NMSS)

From its inception in 1946, the NMSS has enjoyed strong support and guidance from neurologists. This organization, which is largely funded by patient donations, has advocated for MS patients, including guiding the direction of research and funding promising new work. Unfortunately, the first official NMSS response to the new vascular research by Dr. Zamboni was similar to the MS-researcher/neurologist comments previously mentioned: there was little enthusiasm for the vascular approach.

This angered MS patients. One article details this, commenting on MS Society allocation of funds for CCSVI research, then quoting a patient comment regarding these funds: "The society has earmarked $200,000 over two years for research on this procedure. 'That's a joke,' scoffs Katz. The crowd booed at the mention of the MS Society, especially when one protester pointed out it collected $28 million in donations last year" (Green 2010).

MS patients were pleased when the North American NMSS responded to patient outcries for more research funding and announced new grants for CCSVI research; $2.4 million were set aside to investigate CCSVI over several years. However, the initial satisfaction felt by MS patients turned to dismay in June 2010 when they realized the NMSS denied funding to several promising studies proposed by research teams that had publicly supported Dr. Zamboni's new theory.

For example, patients following researchers working to develop this new model expected E. Mark Haacke, PhD's study on iron using a sophisticated type of magnetic resonance called SWI MRI (Haacke 2010b), or David Hubbard, MD's proposal to evaluate MS brains using functional MRI (fMRI), to receive NMSS grants (Hubbard 2010). These studies had proposed to evaluate blood flow in MS patients using more objective methods that are less prone to operator error than ultrasound exams. Such studies would have added to the knowledge base from a different scientific angle by expanding understanding of how occlusions affect blood flow in the brain. Instead, most of the studies that received grants were doppler ultrasound studies headed by MS neurologists/researchers designed to see if people with MS even have venous occlusions.

Some activist patients posting on Internet forums called for a boycott of NMSS activities as a result of what they felt was an underwhelming support of CCSVI research. Others took legal steps to establish new charities with a mission to provide funding for research exclusively on CCSVI, divorcing themselves from the NMSS (Grady 2010). Many activist patients, convinced that CCSVI research was essential, started holding "MStery parties" in their local communities to raise money for CCSVI research. These patient-activists turned to the Internet to get the information they needed in their role as patient advocates and to participate in this growing grassroots movement.

Patient Access to Research

Thomas Freidman says the world is flat (Friedman 2005). By this, he means that the Internet has changed things so that people find themselves on an even playing field concerning access to information. Today, activist groups can obtain formerly exclusive academic information and research.

At one time, specialized knowledge was limited to certain people and others simply did not have access to that information. For instance, if a person needed access to clinical trial results for a new drug, they had to consult certain professionals who were the gatekeepers of that knowledge.

Nowadays, this "flat world" of the Internet has given laypeople access to specialized medical information. In former times, physicians who read about Dr. Zamboni's research in a peer-reviewed journal would have been the only ones to have learned about this revolutionary idea. Researchers would have argued their points in scientific journals as the academic debate moved forward one peer-reviewed paper at a time.

Each phase of research can take several years as one step, particularly in a clinical trial, leads to another. In some cases, researchers must redesign and then restart a study or trial before it can move forward. Conclusive data frequently takes a decade or more to gather as the researchers build the theory study by study.

Thanks to the internet, patients worldwide were talking about Dr. Zamboni's research in MS forums the week it was first released, long before any replication or follow-up studies had been done. Today, such patients continue to watch with avid self-interest as researchers carry out the tedious blow-by-blow process that is scientific debate in literature. These patients are wondering when, and if, they should seek treatment ahead of scientific certainty.

A growing number of physicians and advocates are offering support for the patient who is seeking CCSVI treatment even during its investigational phase. One Canadian oncologist describes this by saying, "An even more important question is what to do right now for symptomatic people with proven neck or chest vein blockage, irrespective of whether they have, or have not, been diagnosed with MS. Based on what we already know about how impaired venous drainage damages other vital organs, as well as the consequences to the central nervous system of sudden jugular vein blockage, should they not be offered immediate treatment under the Canada Health Act?" (Brandes 2010a).

Direct-MS is the second-largest MS charity in Canada. The director of this charity, Ashton Embry, PhD, wrote an open letter to the Canadian Parliament in which he detailed the organization's support for patient treatment:

Most importantly, in the next 10+ years when CCSVI research is being conducted, many people with MS will suffer major, irreversible, increased disability. Any claim that the required research will be done in less than 10 years is not realistic and most MS drugs have taken far longer from start of testing to final approval. Given all of the above, persons with MS do not have the luxury to wait 10 years before gaining access to a treatment which is very safe, reasonably priced and likely very helpful for many [Embry 2010b].

In opposition to this growing advocacy, neurologists have continued to hold a negative stance when interviewed about CCSVI. An MS specialist from Ottawa, Paul Hebert, MD, was quoted as follows:

> "If this were medication we wouldn't be having this discussion" he said, adding that medications are highly regulated and demand rigorous research. "Dr. Zamboni comes around with a novel idea, tries it on 65 people, including his wife, and then it somehow hits the mainstream and everybody advocates for it" [Carlson 2010].

Patients with MS who are interested in CCSVI openly wonder how spokespeople for the neurology community can be so dogmatic and refuse to see any value in evaluating patients for circulatory issues hampering blood flow in the brain. Yet this resistance may be understood in the wider context of modern medicine.

Physicians as Stakeholders

Physicians, along with their primary role, run small businesses. They must meet payroll for an army of billing people to get paid for the work they have done. Medical offices have many hidden costs and are very expensive to run.

Shamefully, insurance companies and Medicare frequently delay reimbursement to physicians, sometimes for months. Compounding the problem, compensation for Medicare services is very poor (Berenson 2010) and less than what is required to keep an office open in many parts of the country; consequently, offices that have a high percentage of Medicare patients (like MS clinics) need to seek alternate forms of income to keep the business afloat. This leaves the physician, who cannot practice his art without being a small businessperson, in a financial bind that can feel very unfair. Indeed, it is unfair.

Neurologists

One alternative form of income that is available to the specialist physician is conducting lectures and seminars to educate other physicians about how to use standard treatments and pharmaceuticals correctly. Pharmaceutical companies compensate doctors for this after-hours work (Lo 2010). This physician/representative becomes expert — a person whose knowledge is deep, with a very good understanding of related research that supports the use of the pharmaceutical compounds he represents.

Other physicians attending these seminars appreciate the opportunity to learn from a leader in the field about how to use the drugs safely. They view this information as the most up-to-date and scientific knowledge available on the subject. Sometimes the pharmaceutical company compensates attendees for attending the seminar as well (Angell 2005, 148).

This situation formalizes endorsement of the current model that guides the use of pharmaceuticals. It generates a feeling that the represented point of view is the only one that exists in the evidence base. This kind of sponsorship of medical education occurs on many levels, from university medical schools to the actual clinician. Some physicians have questioned this arrangement because of the bias it naturally creates (Lo 2010). Marcia Angell, MD, writes extensively about this issue in her well-referenced book *The Truth About Drug Companies: How They Deceive Us and What to Do About It* (Angell 2005, 147).

Commercial advocacy that results from the sponsorship of medical education plays a role in the current discussion. Many specialists in the MS field seem to have lost sight of the fact that there could be previously unrecognized aspects to the disease. Instead, they insist on viewing MS through the narrow lens of autoimmunity. Sponsored medical education is one way the current theory regarding the cause of MS maintains this dominant position.

Clinical trials are another way that the local physician becomes further involved in the current model (Angell 2005, 161). Physicians who run a clinical trial become part of the research team. Their input helps guide the direction of the research (Lo 2010). The physician naturally feels a personal investment in the rationale supporting the trial drug when he runs such a clinical trial.

This rationale is at the very center of the issue. *Rationale* means the medical reasoning and logic that supports the use of the therapy. This reasoning is developed from existing research; this is what is termed the evidence base. Other approaches that are working from the same rationale are not seen as threatening even though they may be market competitors. In fact, these other approaches are just seen as further proof of the value of the rationale.

These twin ways for physicians to be de facto members of the pharmaceutical research industry help to entrench the current treatment model. The point is that MS specialists believe the rationale that drives the pharmaceutical research engine. The majority sincerely think that primary MS autoimmunity is fact, as opposed to theory, and that suppressing immune function is the only possible way to help MS patients.

There is a further perception that everyone agrees these ideas are true and that there is no important evidence opposing the favored rationale. This is false; there is credible research that suggests MS may not be a primary autoimmune disease (see chapter 3).

Nevertheless, the physician tends to put stock in medical literature that affirms the value of pharmaceuticals he can prescribe today that follow the dominant theory regarding the cause of the disorder. When a physician sees research confirming the mainstream view it is considered obviously well-done research, whereas research that offers a new theory may be unfairly critiqued and condemned (Charlton 2008).

Another research team designed a series of experiments to evaluate bias toward a favored position and their findings support the notion that new ideas do not receive fair evaluation:

> This converges with the results from prior studies on sequential information evaluation, in which commitment has been found to be a mediator for the fact that people often fail to revise a hypothesis in accordance with subsequent evidence. As our results imply, not only may they fail to revise their preliminary decision, but they may even actively try to bolster this decision if they focus on it and, thus, feel committed [Jonas et al. 2001].

The authors were evaluating how people commit themselves to one point of view over another and factors that reinforce the commitment. The result of this unconscious selection bias is a belief that all the important research supports the favored point of view. However, there is more than one way to look at a disease. Different specialties see a particular disease from different perspectives.

A fresh look at MS must include vascular specialists at this point in time. They have earned a place at the table.

Vascular Physicians

Many MS patients welcome a new direction of research. This is especially true of people for whom standard therapies are ineffective, and there are many patients in this situation. They do not view the vascular physician as an interloper but rather as an unexpected new resource.

In a live-stream event sponsored by the American Academy of Neurology on April 14, 2010, Dr. Zamboni stated that clinicians ought to consider compassionate treatment for patients with multiple sclerosis if they have exhausted other options (AAN 2010).

Medicine allows any physician to apply his "high degree of clinical suspicion" to patient care, meaning that he is allowed to use his expertise to make a guess that a drug or procedure might work in a situation that it is not approved for because he believes it may help. It is common for neurologists to prescribe a drug never proven to help people with progressive disease out of compassion for such a patient, even if the drug has the potential to cause side effects. Likewise, it is also common for a vascular specialist to apply a known technique to a different, but similar, vascular problem.

The Society of Interventional Radiologists supports their members evaluating patients with MS for CCSVI based on individual circumstances: "When conclusive evidence is lacking, SIR believes that these often difficult decisions are best made by individual patients, their families and their physicians" (SIR 2010).

Angioplasty is an approved technique to repair stenosis in a variety of locations in the body. Using it in a new location is off-label use:

> Although it was, technically, an experimental procedure, Dr. Simon said he did not have to ask his hospital for permission to perform it. The details were similar to other procedures that interventional radiologists do every day. It is not uncommon for them to take a device approved for one purpose and use it for another, like putting a bile-duct stent into a blood vessel — a practice called "off-label" use, which the Food and Drug Administration allows. Interventional radiology, Dr. Simon said, is an "off-label specialty" that depends on innovation and adaptability [Grady 2010].

The vascular community is increasingly speaking out about the value of evaluating blood flow in MS patients. The founder and medical director of the False Creek surgical group in Canada, Mark Godley, MD, stated, "CCSVI exists and it can be treated.... For many MS patients drugs are not working and this is a therapy that needs to be offered to people regardless of whether it is associated with or the root cause of MS" (Godley 2010).

One prominent neurologist advocating for patients in this situation supports separation between clinical treatment and research:

> And I think that in the case of the CCSVI, we should really balance the scientifically rigorous research with respect of the patients' needs and rights, needs to know the results and rights to really grapple with this devastating disease.... But when it comes to diagnostics and treatment, I think this should remain in the domain of the providers. Diagnosis and treatment is not at this time the business of researchers like us who are proceeding on this research [*sic*] [Zivadinov 2010].

Patients understand the principle that good randomized and controlled research must be complete to understand the full scope of the role CCSVI plays in multiple sclerosis. They want researchers to carry out rigorous clinical trials and are seeking ways to support such research.

It might be argued that NMSS fundraisers, such as MS Walks, have long given MS patients a feeling of responsibility toward raising funds for MS research. Patients have been quick to step up and raise funds specifically for CCSVI research — for example, hosting MStery parties and sending the funds raised to Buffalo Neuroimaging Analysis Center (BNAC). The BNAC study is the largest CCSVI study as of this writing, and it has received most of its funding directly from MS patients (Zivadinov 2010). Patients interested in this model want scientific answers and they are willing to pay to get them.

Unfortunately, physicians do not fund studies and they cannot conduct studies without adequate funding. Studies are typically very expensive. The dynamics in the current medical system have put pharmaceutical companies in charge of funding most medical research. This means research with no pharmaceutical potential, like CCSVI, has far fewer resources to tap for funding. Such research frequently suffers from poorly funded studies that are forced to take shortcuts due to lack of funds. The catch-22 is that such studies are frequently panned for being inadequate or "junk science" by proponents of the commercially viable and well-funded model. It also results in an imbalance in the kind of papers that end up comprising the evidence base.

Pharmaceutical Companies as Stakeholders

Pharmaceutical companies earn money for their shareholders and pay their employees by selling medications that they have developed and manufactured. They have a fiduciary responsibility to use their money wisely. That means they make decisions about which research to fund based on both its potential to make the company profitable as well as developing the best drug that will garner the largest market share.

The alternative to corporation-funded research would be to have some kind of publicly funded pharmaceutical research or for the National Multiple Sclerosis Society to fund all research. This is simply not feasible because the cost of developing a new drug is far too great for taxes, MS Walks and donations to support.

Like any company, pharmaceutical companies are interested in their markets. Markets in this case are people with a disease who can be helped by one of their drugs. People with MS do not like to think of themselves as a "market," but that's the way our system works. MS patients need a remedy; the pharmaceutical companies provide it along with the pertinent research.

The pharmaceutical industry has many ways to help people with MS as long as it is widely accepted that multiple sclerosis is caused by problematic immune function alone. MS *is* an inflammatory disease. Inflammation caused by immune system activity is clearly part of the problem, even though it may not be the whole problem. Pharmaceuticals for MS have been proven to reduce symptoms caused by inflammatory immune system activity.

Proponents of the autoimmune model believe there must be a cellular cause for MS, and the research pipeline continues to search for the magic bullet in the immune system that will selectively knock out those cells responsible. The company that can discover such a magic bullet will be able to corner the entire MS pharmaceutical market and will profit greatly. Every company wants to be that company and there is a tremendous amount of money invested in laboratories and personnel to try to find it.

Pharmaceutical companies have become involved in other aspects of the multiple sclerosis community as well. Big, glossy pharmaceutical ads in the NMSS magazine bring revenue into this charitable organization. Patients receive the magazine free of charge and articles often center on the immune system and theoretical mechanisms of autoimmunity in MS. Other points of view are notably missing. For example, there is not a regular column in that magazine on nutritional approaches for MS, although there is a regular section on trials and drugs that are in the research pipeline.

The result of this is that MS patients and their physicians are constantly steeped in a culture that is "primary autoimmune-centric." There is no serious debate on any other modifiable co-factors or different models of MS causation.

Developing an Evidence Base: Politics in Science

The scientific evidence base is critical to good patient care. In chapter 2, the history of MS reveals that for many decades patients were treated based on myth and speculative ideas not supported by science. No one believes it would be beneficial to go back to that way of doing things. However, there is a blind faith that every medical finding is completely objective science and utterly reliable. This is incorrect.

Bias

Bias is a natural human trait and it can influence research. Candace Pert, PhD, the scientist who discovered the opiate mu receptor, said in a lecture that people have an idea that science is "this big objective thing" but in reality scientists know what they're looking for before they begin, and they design their experiment to prove what they already think is true. She talks about how she designed an experiment but did not find the cannabinoid receptor she was looking for. She conducted many experiments in which she did not find a cannabinoid receptor, but she "knew" one had to be there. Eventually someone else found it. That person also "knew" it had to be there (Pert 2000).

The problem comes when the expected assumption is not proven. When conclusive research has not been completed, innate belief cannot substitute for proof.

Group Bias

Group mentality is different from individual mentality. When there is a group, individuals tend to go along with the majority opinion rather than point out areas where they might disagree. Medical specialties are powerful groups.

A paper published by Charlton in 2008 titled "False, Trivial, Obvious: Why New and Revolutionary Theories Are Typically Disrespected" discusses the dynamics that serve to suppress new ideas in medical science. The people subscribing to the current dogma typically vigorously reject a new idea as false. As work continues on the new idea, it goes through a stage in which it is accepted as true but trivial. In the current debate, this might be an attitude of "yes, we agree there are venous stenoses, but they do not matter." The final stage in the evolution of a new idea is acceptance, wherein everyone agrees the new idea is obviously true (Charlton 2008).

Marian Simka suggested in a published comment on the article above that it may be possible for new ideas to skip the first stage by purposefully presenting the new idea as true but unimportant to the current model's position as prime driver of the disease process from the beginning (Simka 2008). There are actually politics in science.

GROUP BIAS STUDIED • In 1987 sociologists Malcolm Nicolson and Cathleen McLaughlin from London published a paper on social constructionism and MS theory. They were evaluating the dynamics related to the ways in which a favored medical opinion comes to predominate. "Constructionism" is a concept describing the ways that people generate knowledge and meaning from their beliefs and experiences (preconceived notions) and not strictly from what is real and happening around them.

The published paper discussed how groups of people with different ideas about the cause of multiple sclerosis interact. The opposing models chosen by the authors to evaluate these dynamics were a vascular theory, which proposed that tiny fat embolisms cause obstruction of small blood vessels in the brain, and the standard autoimmune theory of MS. The physicians who were advocating this particular vascular theory focused on features of MS that suggest a vascular component plays a role in the disease. The fat embolism idea was a hypothesis to explain these vascular features.

This historical "vascular versus autoimmune" debate occurred during the early 1980s and was part of a wider debate about whether hyperbaric oxygen was useful in MS. The authors of the paper on social constructionism point out that the autoimmune proponents were the dominant group (Nicolson and McLaughlin 1987).

Immunology as a field was considered especially prestigious and this gave their point of view an advantage. The authors of the paper cited above stated:

> However it should also be noted that in such contexts as this — where distinctions between valid and invalid medical knowledge must be made — questions of expertise interconnect with questions of power. Immunology has possession of the commanding heights of Orthodox medicine (Humphrey 1982) and accordingly possesses great power — power to grant recognition, to open access to publication, to fund research. Moreover neurologists and immunologists have always dominated the medical advisory committees of the British and American multiple sclerosis societies, major grant givers in the field of MS research. The debate over causation and treatment of MS is not, therefore, an interchange of ideas between social equals, but is a competition between a large and powerful social group and a weak and a marginal one [Nicolson and McLaughlin 1987].

People generally assume that medicine is based on scientific standards. Many individuals presumably believe that if a scientific experiment is legitimate and the findings are important, the medical community will naturally accept the findings.

However, in the study evaluating constructionism in science, the dominant group repeatedly rejected studies showing any value in using hyperbaric oxygen as if they were meaningless. Even positive findings were rejected and studies with such findings were dismissed as being poorly done or in some other way invalid. The dominant groups, immunology and neurology, set the ground rules for how to evaluate multiple sclerosis, and observations with their basis in vascular facts were treated as insignificant information.

Nicolson and McLaughlin document that the *New England Journal of Medicine* (NEJM) published a double-blind placebo-controlled trial on hyperbaric oxygen, which showed a 75 percent improvement in participating MS patients. The same issue published a trial on cyclophosphamide (an immunosuppressant). The cyclophosphamide trial was not double-blind or placebo-controlled; the results showed an improvement in one third of trial participants and stabilization in an additional one third.

Nicolson and McLaughlin concluded that from a purely scientific standpoint, the more compelling study should have been hyperbaric oxygen (HBO). The HBO trial had better scientific design, patients responded more positively, and it is the safer of the two approaches. In spite of this, the NEJM editors commented that the cyclophosphamide trial further affirmed that MS is an autoimmune disease and that this was a very positive note for MS research. They commented, on the other hand, that the trial on hyperbaric oxygen showed "much less impressive results." Nicolson and McLaughlin even document that the chairman of the medical advisory committee of the NMSS stated plainly that he simply "did not believe" the HBO research (Nicolson and McLaughlin 1987).

The debate about hyperbaric oxygen in MS was eventually dropped. Interested researchers could not get funding and the few positive studies were not substantial enough to be conclusive. A recent Cochrane review of the subject concluded, "The small number of analyses suggestive of benefit are isolated, difficult to ascribe with biological plausibility and would need to be confirmed in future well-designed trials. Such trials are not, in our view, justified by this review" (Bennett and Heard 2004).

By commenting "difficult to ascribe with biological plausibility," the reviewers are indicating that they do not believe the vascular hypothesis and therefore positive findings are suspect in their view. Yet seen from a different perspective the approach plausibly has value if MS turns out to be a type of venous disease; according to researchers investigating chronic venous disease in legs, HBO modestly improves oxygenation and healing in lesions caused by venous insufficiency (Ulkur et al. 2002).

In a repeat of the dynamics seen in the 1980s, in 2010, the proponents of the current standard of treatment have mischaracterized the Italian researchers' published body of work as one single study, as if that is all there is underpinning this new model (Blackwell 2010; Carlson 2010). Another author claimed there were severe ethical problems with the research from Italy, stating that "few, if any, ethics committees would approve conducting experiments at such an early stage" (Corcoran 2010). This comment ignored the fact that an ethics committee had approved the study in question, precisely because the research was past the early stage and the series of earlier studies justified a new study that included procedures. Another group argued that the new hypothesis was implausible based on the current widely accepted model, as if any other hypothesis is invalid by virtue of the fact that it is not based on the dominant model (Krogias et al. 2010).

Today's debate is also similar in that some articles in the medical literature suggest that factors other than autoimmunity play a role in MS, yet these published works continue to be largely invisible as part of the debate about MS causation. One could argue that there is a power structure, and that social constructionism plays a role in establishing the dominant theory even in a scientific field.

Necessity of Trials

Randomized controlled trials (RCTs) that are also blinded are the gold standard for proving the safety and efficacy of new treatments. Controlled means that some of the people in the trial receive the treatment the researchers are testing and others receive either a placebo or treatment with known efficacy for comparison. Randomized means that the researchers randomly assigned the trial participants to one of these groups. When the trial is single-blinded then either the people in the trial or the researchers do not know which treatment individual people received; when it's double-blinded neither the researchers nor the people know which treatment they received. Medicine takes great pride in the evidence generated by the blinded RCT because it removes bias; by making sure researchers and patients are not aware of which treatment they received, the findings reliably reflect the true value of the therapy rather than belief about its value.

However, this type of trial is not best for all situations. The RCT is best when researchers can give trial participants exactly the same treatment. This is true when researchers want to test a new drug because the drug given to each trial participant in the treatment arm is identical. However, when the treatment is a procedure and still in the discovery phase, observational research moves science forward more quickly.

Researchers use the observational approach when discovery is the more important aspect of the work (Vandenbroucke 2008). The discovery phase of a new model is necessary when physicians do not yet fully understand the new problem and its treatment. Observational studies allow the researcher to notice something unexpected and then change treatment for the next trial participant to incorporate the new discovery. Once the researcher fully understands the new treatment, he can design an RCT with confidence.

Observational studies are more common in surgical treatments and procedures like angioplasty. The reason is that the clinician doing the procedure is not certain yet of the details involved — what exactly to look for and how to best repair the area. In this case, if an RCT is done before the operator is experienced, he becomes what is known in scientific circles as a confounding factor; if the treatment failed the researcher does not know if the failure was because the model was wrong or if the operator did not yet have the skill and experience to be effective.

Treatment for CCSVI is currently in the discovery phase (see chapter 6). Once discovery is complete and there are physicians experienced in assessment and treatment of CCSVI, they can teach others. Randomized controlled trials based on those refined approaches will eventually make clear which procedures are best for the different kinds of problems that patients with CCSVI present, as well as clarifying the impact effective, well-done treatment has on MS.

Researchers can design RCTs when they understand all of the different occlusions associated with CCSVI and how to treat them. Vascular researchers working toward finding these answers have produced an impressive number of studies and data in a relatively short period (see chapters 5 and 6). However, until the discovery process is complete and vascular specialists have defined standardized treatment protocols, it should be understood that CCSVI treatment may or *may not* be effective for a given individual (see chapter 6).

Researchers must discover other aspects as well, such as whether CCSVI causes MS or if CCSVI merely worsens MS. It may also be present in healthy people, suggesting that the presence of CCSVI alone does not cause MS and other factors are at work. The effectiveness of treatment of these stenoses will remain unknown until the full range of comparative research is complete. Both vascular specialists, who must be the researchers to define how best to discover and treat these vascular malformations, and neurologists, who must be the ones to define how the best treatment affects multiple sclerosis, need to be involved in order for research to be comprehensive.

Quackery and Snake Oil

Each of the various stakeholders mentioned in this chapter sincerely believes that they are doing the best possible thing for all people involved. The CEOs of pharmaceutical companies talk about their commitment to further research on promising new scientific approaches that have commercial potential, both to help MS patients and to grow their corporations. The medical director of the NMSS is quoted in interviews talking about how the newest pharmaceutical approaches are thought to be a breakthrough for MS patients (AAN 2010, 4). MS researchers are genuinely looking for solutions and believe that they are designing significant research.

Physicians who believe in the current paradigm have invested countless hours and years of their lives helping to develop the autoimmune model. They believe they are on the right track and are anxious to defend and protect vulnerable MS patients from quackery and poor science (Samson 2010). Unfortunately, there's been a lot of that.

MS history is riddled with many failed hypotheses. Recent years have seen an irrational exuberance over bee-sting therapy, yeast, and various foods either as a healing food or the culprit food, fats either as a key to good health or as a culprit, raw foods and sometimes even kooky procedures; a fellow gym member once told the author of this book that colonics would cure MS!

Proponents of the fads often justify their approach by combing the literature for papers that they might reinterpret as support for their theory. Such reinterpretation oversteps scientific bounds because it implies the original research evaluated factors or substances it was never designed to evaluate. The result is that these ideas fool vulnerable patients into thinking there is scientific support for the new idea that does not exist. This kind of pseudo-science can sound very convincing.

The problem is when people try to pretend that Dr. Zamboni's research fits into this category in order to marginalize the findings. In contrast to fads, there has been evidence of a vascular component in multiple sclerosis for 170 years, although technology in prior decades was inadequate for meaningful evaluation. Not even contemporary neurologists deny there is a vascular element to MS; their point of view is simply that the vascular features of MS are an *epiphenomenon* (side issue unrelated to cause) and not relevant to the MS process. Also in contrast to fads, the modern-day research on CCSVI is based on good peer-reviewed research designed specifically to evaluate cerebrospinal blood flow in MS patients, although people do need to exercise caution in interpreting early findings.

The Internet is a natural ally for the MS patient in regard to advancing understanding about CCSVI among patients.

What Happened on the Internet

As mentioned at the beginning of this chapter, the Internet gives MS patients access to medical information. Resources like PubMed, the National Institutes of Health searchable database of published medical literature, and Google Scholar give MS patients resources that weren't available in the past. Today, new peer-reviewed published medical research is available at the nearest computer.

Some online forums cater to people who are interested in reading and discussing new scientific papers. One such online forum is ThisIsMS.com, referred to as TIMS by members. Each chapter of this book begins with a quote posted on TIMS by an MS patient in relation to the debate on CCSVI and MS.

The TIMS online community has been up and running since 2003. There are TIMS members who believe MS is autoimmune, and members who believe MS is primarily degenerative. Discussions sometimes get heated as people argue their point in cyber-debates. There are also separate forums on TIMS for people taking each of the drugs approved for MS. It is a vital community about all things MS. TIMS is not sponsored by any commercial interest, nor is the content censored in any way. Members love it.

One member, "Dignan," has maintained a thread for several years in which he keeps track of new drug trials and research in the pipeline. Dignan posted a link to Dr. Zamboni's third study evaluating patients with MS for CCSVI in December 2008.

This paper held special significance for another forum member, "Cheerleader," whose favored theory about MS causation was that endothelial dysfunction (essentially a leaky blood-brain barrier) is the root cause of multiple sclerosis. Cheerleader was very excited when Dr. Zamboni's paper came out because its premise fit neatly with her own belief.

Cheerleader, whose real name is Joan Beal and whose husband is the MS patient in their family, started an exclusive thread for CCSVI-focused discussion. Ideas early on were full of misconceptions as forum members grappled with trying to learn and understand the new theory. People who had been thinking about and discussing MS in terms of immunology suddenly struggled to understand vascular physiology. Members discussed literature related to venous disease as well as how nutrients such as vitamin D insufficiency might relate to this issue.

Joan, who has the soul of a community organizer, coupled with a sincere heart, repeatedly encouraged other forum members to contact the vascular department at their local university for evaluation of blood flow. There was an air of excitement and hope among TIMS members that possibly someone's local university would take a look at this research and get involved because a member brought it to their attention. Many members were willing to pay out of pocket to be examined with duplex ultrasonography as recommended by Dr. Zamboni, just to try to hurry along awareness and research at the local level.

The first forum member to find a physician willing to perform the testing was "Cure-or-bust," an Aussie fondly called "Cure" online. A physician evaluated Cure using color Doppler ultrasound and identified one abnormal parameter. However, the physician was disappointed and called the evaluation a failure when he did not see two abnormal parameters, as Dr. Zamboni's research predicted he should.

The second forum member to locate a physician willing to perform the testing was the author of this book. This test revealed reflux in my vertebral veins. The vascular specialist I consulted considered it interesting, but not treatable because the vertebral veins are small (this physician's initial interpretation turned out to be incomplete — there were other blockages that were causing the vertebral vein reflux). My personal account, along with other patients' experiences, is described in more detail in chapter 7.

The third person to be tested was Joan's husband Jeff. Joan hit a home run when she contacted Michael Dake, MD, of the Falk Cardiovascular Center at Stanford University and introduced him to Dr. Zamboni's research along with an impassioned plea to test her husband. Dr. Dake was initially skeptical, but after evaluating the research and a consultation with Dr. Zamboni at a symposium where each happened to be presenting research papers, he realized the idea had merit.

Testing ordered by Dr. Dake for Jeff included not only a Doppler exam but also magnetic resonance venography (MRV), and transverse MRI of the neck. These last two imaging procedures are different tests from those Dr. Zamboni typically uses, but in Jeff's case they were essential for diagnosis. Jeff's standard Doppler exam showed nothing unusual. However, the MRV and MRI clearly showed gross stenosis of both internal jugular veins with occlusions at 90 percent and extensive collateral circulation.

As a result, Dr. Dake offered his opinion that stenoses such as these could be repaired, although he had no idea if such a repair would have any impact on the disease course in MS. It seemed plausible that Jeff's severe headaches and some other symptoms were related to this vascular defect because venous occlusions (like superior vena cava syndrome or jugular occlusion) cause symptoms similar to what Jeff was experiencing and are conditions that must be treated. For this reason, Jeff decided to have his stenoses repaired.

A venogram followed by angioplasty and stents if needed was scheduled for the next day. The venogram confirmed the stenosis seen on MRV and was followed by placement of bilateral stents during the same procedure. Jeff had immediate feelings of clear-headedness and a lifting of the heavy congested feeling he had come to experience as normal. The headaches cleared up. Within a few days, it was clear that his fatigue had dissipated and he no longer napped during the day. He was suddenly able to work full days and even began engaging in evening social activities again, something he had not done for several years.

Joan shared details of the treatment with the online community. Dr. Dake was soon flooded with requests for evaluation as patients drafted him into service. He had to hire a dedicated receptionist to handle this sudden workload, eventually treating 46 people in observational study before he moved to an actual institutional review board (IRB) approved trial.

Most of the patients who initially saw Dr. Dake were members of TIMS and the vast majority of them reported that Dr. Dake saw evidence of stenosis when he did venograms. Patients realized some form of database would be helpful so members could see how treated people recovered after the procedure. Members started a tracking thread in which the treated members could record their anecdotal results for everyone else to see. The thread still exists today for interested readers at ThisIsMS.com.

Other members of TIMS were energized and enthusiastic about these findings. People began to pursue physicians in their local communities who would consider evaluating patients.

"Bestadmom," a New Yorker who wanted treatment in her own community, sent out 250 letters to local physicians searching for someone who would evaluate her. She discovered an interventional radiologist on the East Coast who agreed to treat several people as an observational study.

Online, forum members shared approaches that seemed effective in helping them find physicians to evaluate them at local clinics. Other forum members then tried the same methods. As a result, online patients have managed to recruit a growing number of physicians around the United States, and indeed around the world, to be part of this new paradigm, all thanks to patient activism and doctors who are open-minded enough to listen.

Joan's advocacy for her husband and her sharing of their experience online grew organically into a grassroots movement that has spread to many countries. As information rolls in from clinical vascular doctors everywhere, it is clear that the vast majority of MS patients appear to have CCSVI. It will be some years before the extent of CCSVI's contribution to MS pathology is known. In the meantime, many patients are seeking clinics where they can get evaluation and treatment, if it is indicated (see chapter 6).

As a result of interaction on the Internet, this "flat world" has changed the dynamic significantly in the politics of medicine. Many patients refuse to be left out of the ongoing conversation. For the first time MS patients have demanded in an activist effort that the medical community hear their voices.

There are some people who find themselves suddenly not knowing how they fit in this new arrangement. They express concerns that perhaps this could mean the end of good, rigorous evidence-based healthcare. They would like to reframe this debate so that it is seen as a debate about science, as if scientific principles themselves are being attacked and tossed aside by a populace too naïve to understand what they demand (Carlson 2010).

However, it could be argued that commercial interests have long held the evidence base captive (Giles 2006). There is credible research in the evidence base that questions the idea that MS is purely an autoimmune disease. In spite of this, clinicians treat patients based solely on that model every day as if such research does not exist.

Today, there is suddenly important research and vast anecdotal evidence, including that from clinicians, that indicates MS has a vascular component. Where are the voices that demand discussion of this evidence? They are patient voices.

2

Multiple Sclerosis:
History and Epidemiology

People see what they are prepared to see — posted on TIMS

The medical literature, with its wealth of evidence-based medicine, is a tremendously rich resource. There are curious researchers all over the world trying to solve the riddle of MS, and there have been for many decades.

Dr. Zamboni's new research does not negate prior research; it brings to light a component of MS that simply had not been appreciated. Understanding the vascular model may clarify a previously invisible factor that plays a role in the actual disease process that is multiple sclerosis. Looking at the evidence base in this light may reveal how these two potential factors of multiple sclerosis, immune and vascular, may interact.

This chapter looks at the history and epidemiology of multiple sclerosis. It lays special emphasis on those published works that might clarify how a vascular component to MS may have been missed.

Multiple Sclerosis: A Brief Overview

MS is the most common cause of neurological disability in young adults. It is most often diagnosed between the ages of 20 and 50, though there are occasional atypical cases diagnosed outside this usual time frame.

Today MS is typically diagnosed using magnetic resonance imaging, or MRI. With this technology it is possible to see areas that show an abnormal signal in comparison to healthy brain tissue. These "bright spots" visible on MRI may be an excess of fluid in the tissue or may represent older scar tissue. The radiologist recognizes these changes as diagnostic for MS when seen on an MRI.

Bright spots seen on MRI often appear and disappear in scans of MS patients' brains when done on a regular basis. The MS patient who feels well often has this MRI evidence of new MS activity even though they have no new symptoms. This suggests MS damage is an ongoing process even when people are in remission with no obvious disease activity.

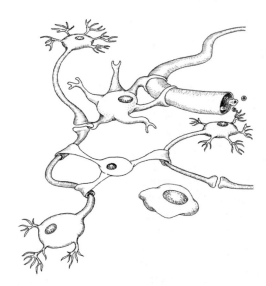

This drawing shows the cells of the brain. A blood vessel is shown in the upper right corner; there is a star-shaped astrocyte attached to the blood vessel and it is also stretching over on the other side to the gap between two nerve cells. Astrocytes are the most plentiful cell type in the brain and fill the spaces between the nerves; they provide support functions for the other cells of the brain, including maintenance of the blood-brain barrier (which is why it is attached to the blood vessel), supplying nutrients to the nerve cells, and repair and scarring after cell damage. There are three nerves depicted in this image; the fat part of the nerve with the branched arms is called the cell body and the long part that reaches over to the next nerve is called the axon. The signal goes from nerve to nerve down the axons until it triggers the target function. The oligodendrocyte, just below the astrocyte near the center, is myelinating the axons of two nerve cells. Nerve cells do not make their own myelin, the oligodendrocytes do it for them. If a nerve loses its myelin, an oligodendrocyte can make new myelin. If the oligodendrocytes are lost altogether in one area, this will cause permanent demyelination. There is a microglia, the brain's resident immune system cell similar to a macrophage, below the oligodendrocyte. Image courtesy of Marv Miller.

A *clinically silent lesion* is the term for a lesion that is visible on MRI but does not have corresponding new symptoms. It is clear that MS lesion activity is far more frequent than the patient is aware; silent lesions outnumber clinical relapses by as much as 10 to 1 (Bjartmer and Trapp 2001).

The term *clinical relapse* refers to a relapse that results in a loss of function noticeable to the patient — a suddenly paralyzed hand or loss of vision, for example. Such a relapse is also called an attack or exacerbation.

"Lesions that are inflammatory and demyelinating in nature" cause these relapses (McDonald 2001). This explanation of a relapse describes the pathological changes seen in the MS brain when it is examined during an autopsy.

Tissue in the active MS

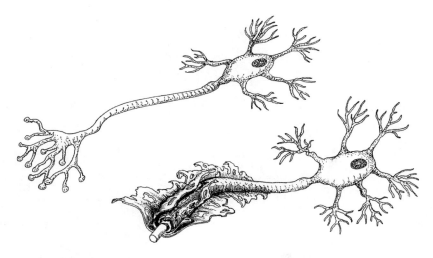

This image shows a healthy nerve cell with intact myelin and a demyelinated axon. (The oligodendrocyte, which is responsible for creating myelin, is not depicted in this image.) A demyelinated nerve cannot carry nerve signals properly and therefore the associated body function is lost because the signal spills out and doesn't reach the next nerve cell. Image courtesy of Marv Miller.

lesion is inflamed with obvious immune system activity. This means that there is additional fluid in the area and many cells of the immune system are actively working on the tissue. The oligodendrocytes and the myelin made by them appear to be the primary cells damaged, resulting in the descriptive term *demyelination*.

Nerves with no myelin lose their ability to function correctly. This causes the acute clinical relapse. When a new oligodendrocyte (cell that produces myelin) moves in and reinsulates the nerve with a fresh coating of myelin, its corresponding function returns. The patient then experiences what is termed a *remission*, meaning they are back to functioning normally or near normally.

These events primarily occur in the white matter of the brain. There is also degeneration, which is not readily visible on MRI, in the gray matter. It appears that inflammation and demyelination are the causes of short-term losses in function, while long-term progressive changes are due to degeneration of the nerves themselves.

MS Patterns

People with the diagnosis of MS do not all experience the disease in the same way. There are different classifications of MS, and each has a pattern of symptoms unique to that group. It is not known if these are simply differences in symptom pattern or actual differences in disease subtype.

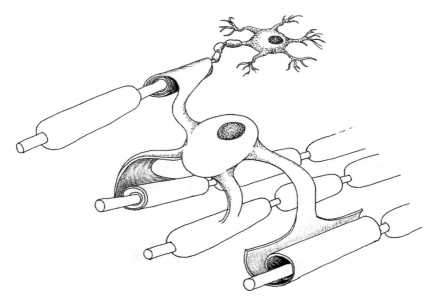

In this image an oligodendrocyte is remyelinating the axons of four cells that had previously lost myelin in a relapse. Remyelination allows nerve signals to move down the axon properly and the corresponding body function returns, triggering remission. Sometimes the remyelinating oligodendrocyte is a new one and sometimes it is a nearby cell that reaches over to repair the demyelinated area. Image courtesy of Marv Miller.

Relapsing remitting multiple sclerosis, or RRMS, is the most common pattern. Roughly 85 percent of MS patients experience RRMS. It is characterized by relapses that remit (go away). Relapses caused by inflammatory demyelination naturally diminish over time in people with RRMS so that fewer relapses over the years are the norm (Murray 2005, 328).

Eventually, most people with RRMS convert to what is termed secondary progressive multiple sclerosis (SPMS), wherein there is continual loss of function with no noticeable relapses. There may be no inflammation seen on MRI during this phase of the illness, but degeneration causes loss of tissue in the brain and atrophy.

In primary progressive MS, or PPMS, the person accumulates progressive losses of function or disability with no relapse or remission from the beginning of the disease. Primary progressive patients gain disability more rapidly overall than RRMS patients do.

Benign disease is a less-often-diagnosed pattern in which the person remains stable for many years. Exacerbations tend to remit entirely.

Advanced diagnostics of modern medicine were not available to early researchers, yet they documented important physical characteristics that are pertinent to today's debate regarding potential venous involvement with MS pathology. In the next section, the history of MS will be reviewed with a special emphasis on facts that might relate to the venous model.

History of Multiple Sclerosis

In 1863 Dr. E. Rindfleisch was doing an autopsy of a person who had had MS. He noted:

> If one looks carefully at freshly altered parts of the white matter ... one perceives already with the naked eye a red point or line in the middle of each individual focus ... the lumen of a small vessel engorged with blood.... All this leads us to search for the primary cause of the disease in an alteration of individual vessels and their ramifications; All vessels running inside the foci, but also those which traverse the immediately surrounding but still intact parenchyma are in a state characteristic of chronic inflammation [Rindfleisch 1863].

Dr. Rindfleisch considered the blood vessel anomaly an important clue to the disease that required more investigation.

Scattered earlier findings came together in Jean-Martin Charcot. People refer to this curious physician as the "father of neurology" because his interest in the brain and scientific methods would be the model that later researchers in the field would follow. His insistence on the verifiable rather than the supposed was a leap forward in medical thought at a time when myth and old wives' tales were commonly employed in medical care.

Charcot's drawings of autopsy findings in patients who died of MS clearly show the hardened sclerotic plaques in the brain and spinal cord, as well as the widened perivascular spaces noted by previous workers. Charcot felt that the more important question regarding the changes in the blood vessels was what caused them to be that way, assuming their changes were a result of MS rather than the cause of it (Murray 2005, 118).

The differing opinions of Rindfleisch and Charcot regarding whether the vascular changes were a result or the cause of MS would remain largely unsettled in the minds of physicians all the way through the 1950s.

In 1870 Louis Ranvier discovered myelin. This important discovery revealed that the myelin coating on the nerves is the factor that allows the nerve to function correctly. Myelin on the nerve functions like the rubber coating on the wires of an electrical cord; it keeps the electrical impulse moving down the nerve and not spilling out, which would weaken the signal. Understanding this was an important milestone for MS because loss of myelin is the hallmark of the disease.

In 1884 Pierre Marie put forth the idea that multiple sclerosis was an infectious disease. Among his findings regarding MS lesions was the fact that there were blood clots adhering to the walls in the small vessels (Schelling 2004, 70). These blood clots were seen as part of the infective process and not as a venous issue. The idea that some kind of infective agent plays a role in MS would periodically gain steam over the following decades as researchers uncovered new information in the field of infectious disease. Even today's authors mention the possibility that an infective agent is the cause of MS (Hemmer et al. 2002).

In 1916 James Dawson described MS lesions in detail. This included the fact that in the center of each lesion was an inflamed vein. On the microscopic scale Dr. Dawson noted that oligodendrocytes were damaged and dying (Barnett et al. 2006).

Scientific methods became more available through the mid-century. The discovery of experimental autoimmune encephalomyelitis (EAE) and the creation of the National Multiple Sclerosis Society (NMSS) caused this shift, as discussed in the next section.

The Immune System vs. Vascular Causes

In 1935 Thomas Rivers discovered that injecting foreign brain proteins into an animal caused what was thought to be a type of allergic reaction in the brain. This reaction included inflammation, demyelination, and subsequent paralysis, though the disease was self-limited, meaning it ended on its own and the animal recovered. However, this was important for MS research because the demyelination was similar to that seen in MS; it was thought that researchers would be able to create a true animal version of multiple sclerosis by refining the technique.

The development of a reliable EAE model, which would be useful for studying multiple sclerosis, took place over the course of a decade. By 1949 Peter Olitsky and Robert Yager were able to induce acute disseminated encephalomyelitis in mice, establishing the mouse form of EAE (Lavi and Constantinescu 2005, 11).

Experimentally inducing EAE made it possible to scientifically study these animals and test theories in a controlled lab setting. While MS and EAE are not the same disease, the demyelination was similar enough that researchers viewed this animal model as an important step forward. The differences between these two diseases and how they affect MS research will be discussed in more depth in chapter 3.

An entirely different line of scientific inquiry into the cause of MS emerged during the same time frame in which the animal model EAE was being developed. A neurologist named Tracy Putnam was working on the theory that a problem in the vascular system caused multiple sclerosis.

During the period from 1931 through 1936 Dr. Putnam did experiments on dogs in which he occluded the blood vessels leading from the brain to observe what happened to surrounding brain tissue. These experiments on dogs were designed to test the idea that occlusion (blockage) of the veins was the cause of MS.

Dr. Putnam caused *encephalopathy* (pathological changes in the brain) in the dogs when he occluded their veins. Critics identified this animal model as a form of acute disseminated encephalitis rather than experimental MS. However, Dr. Putnam continued to pursue this line of work and countered that as the venous occlusion was left in place, older lesions developed into typical representations of MS lesions. He stated that the lesions were so similar to MS lesions that a similar mechanism must cause MS (Putnam 1935). Dr. Putnam published a number of papers on his research based on his venous model. He believed blocked veins, either an occlusion or blood clots, caused MS (Swiderski 1998, 136).

Dr. Putnam continued to follow this path of inquiry and in 1942 gave a speech at the American Medical Association in which he stated MS was due to faulty blood clotting. In his view, this was the initial event that started the changes that eventually result in the clinical picture of MS.

There was no diagnostic test at that time able to evaluate the venous blood flow in living people or animals. Venography was not available until 1967. In the 1940s there was no way for Dr. Putnam to fully evaluate the blood flow in humans diagnosed with MS.

In August 1946 Dr. Putnam announced the results of his trial on MS patients using the blood thinner dicoumarin. The results were not as promising as hoped, though Putnam continued to use the drug in patients with MS to help reduce exacerbations (Swiderski 1998, 158). Coincidentally, this was the year the sister of an MS patient founded the National Multiple Sclerosis Society (NMSS). Tracy Putnam was one of 20 neurologists who became the original physician members of the NMSS.

Dr. Putnam took the opportunity to present the vascular theory of MS causation when the NMSS gave him a chance to head a committee that published a manual for physicians about the disease. This was the first project tackled by the NMSS: the goal was to create access to information for physicians throughout the country so patients would get consistent, modern care. Because of the manual, the vascular cause of MS was widely accepted in the 1950s.

An interesting study by Richard Brickner in 1953 detailed the use of amyl nitrite, a vasodilator, on patients in the midst of a relapse. It was discovered in the early 1950s that this medication caused reversal of symptoms in moments. Here is a quote from the paper: "Relief of the fresh phenomena occurs repeatedly and predictably within a few minutes of the vasodilation" (Brickner 1953).

The paper goes on to state that though it was well known that vasodilators cause relief of relapse symptoms, these changes appeared to be temporary. The vasodilators caused an acute "flush," during which relapse symptoms would suddenly abate, only to return to pretreatment levels afterward. The point of this paper was to discuss the use of this drug in a regimen that hopefully would result in longer-lasting improvements.

The authors gave periodic doses of the vasodilator over several days to three patients having an acute relapse. They reported each administration of the drug caused more, longer-lasting relief until finally the symptoms did not recur, and the patient returned to pre-relapse levels of function (Brickner 1953). This seemed to be effective only for relapses; it was not helpful in progressive disease. This tiny study was very limited but it suggested that poor blood flow contributes to MS relapse symptoms.

Another approach used in the 1950s to dilate the blood vessels was histamine given intravenously. Hinton Jonez used it on 1,500 patients with apparent success (Jonez 1952). Dr. Jonez died and his work seems to have died along with him as the mainstream medical community did not develop this work, though today some alternative practitioners offer a histamine-based product, Prokarin (EDMS, LLC), as a helpful complementary adjunct to standard therapy.

Vascular approaches and available therapeutic approaches in the 1940s and 1950s were very limited. As mentioned, Dr. Putnam used blood thinners based on his modest success in human trials. In addition, vasodilators like amyl nitrite and histamine were used in trials with some success, but these approaches from isolated clinical studies were not widely adopted. Unfortunately, in the wider medical community such unscientific devices as the "circulation stimulator" were also used on MS patients with no clinical support or trial whatsoever (Rolak 2009).

MS Research Becomes More Scientific

In the years between 1930 and 1960 strides were made toward the development of modern MS research. In 1934 the American Neurological Association outlined a protocol to standardize clinical trials including randomization and controls. This was in response to literally hundreds of bizarre treatments, each tried on a few patients with vague parameters for success. Such research could not provide useful information for the general MS population due to these limitations. Dr. Putnam did a meta-analysis of such studies and declared that 49 percent of 1,407 patients treated in these trials improved; meanwhile, 69 percent of 133 untreated patients got better (McAlpine and Compston 2006, 64)!

Treating patients based on scientific findings became a realistic goal as quality research began to be produced. The divergence of the vascular and immunological theories regarding MS development occurred during this time. The budding field of immunology was off to a promising start, offering sophisticated techniques and ways to test hypotheses in an objective, scientific manner through the observation of animals with EAE. Small manageable animals like mice and guinea pigs were the perfect solution for investigating scientific questions.

Human MS is so variable that it is difficult to define success in patients receiving experimental treatment with consistency without also making an effort to control for numerous factors. In contrast, there are few "mouse variables" to control so findings in EAE reliably quantify what the researcher is investigating.

In contrast, the unsophisticated vascular technologies of the time, lack of useful vascular diagnostics to gauge success, and lack of clear success using limited drugs of the day all worked together to lend a "been there, done that" attitude to vascular theories as a cause of MS.

The vascular model was largely abandoned by the late 1950s and research became focused around the animal model.

MS History Marches On

In 1947, just a year after the NMSS was founded, a researcher named Elvin Kabat developed a cerebrospinal fluid test for detecting the presence of oligoclonal bands. Dr. Kabat's research seemed to confirm the immune model of MS causation. Oligoclonal bands are evidence of immune activity.

In 1960 the very first controlled trial of a drug for the treatment of MS was completed. This was a trial on the adrenocorticotropic hormone, or ACTH. This drug causes the adrenal gland to make corticosteroids. MS researchers viewed this as further confirmation that the theory of immune causation was probably correct because steroids aggressively suppress immune activity.

In the 1980s it was discovered that it is possible for the immune system to mistakenly attack self tissue after infection with a virus. This finding would generate the hypothesis that some type of viral trigger is the starting point for autoimmune activation in MS. It was also discovered that it is the macrophage, an immune system cell that breaks down tissue, which is present in the damaged areas of the MS brain.

Scientific research was building a huge evidence base of objective findings that seemed to keep circling back to immune function. Researchers gradually forgot about other ideas and began to see EAE as essentially the same as MS.

MRI and EDSS: Groundbreaking Tools for Research

Magnetic resonance imaging (MRI) was discovered in 1981. The diagnosis of MS in 1970 took, on average, seven years. The use of MRI has reduced to that time to six months. MRI also caused an impressive growth in what was known about MS, shattering long-held beliefs.

Using MRI it was discovered that clinically silent lesions in MS greatly outnumber the lesions that cause physical symptoms and relapses. This finding established that there is not actually a "remission" from the standpoint of the brain, resulting in an important shift in thinking about MS. Physicians no longer consider remissions periods of no disease activity. This fact is why many neurologists encourage patients to start on a disease-modifying drug (DMD) soon after diagnosis. The saying "time is brain" used by neurologists reflects the fact that every day brain cells are lost to the MS process.

A milestone was reached in 1983 when Dr. John Kurtzke designed the expanded disability severity score (EDSS) for evaluating symptoms in MS. For the first time, researchers could consistently quantify changes in an MS patient's functional level for comparison. An EDSS of 0 is defined as a completely functional person and an EDSS of 10 defines death from multiple sclerosis.

With the introduction of the EDSS, patients could be objectively assessed to see how they were progressing or responding to therapeutic interventions. This made it possible for researchers to evaluate patient function in a consistent and meaningful way.

The MRI gave researchers a way to examine changes in the brain while a patient was living. This significantly changed understanding of the MS disease process. Coupled with the EDSS, researchers now had the tools needed to assess potential pharmaceutical approaches. This laid the groundwork for a pharmaceutical boom.

Pharmaceuticals Arrive for MS Patients

In the 1990s pharmaceuticals specifically designed for multiple sclerosis would finally be available after decades of research. In 1993 the first drug for multiple sclerosis was introduced; it was an interferon.

Interferons were discovered in the 1950s. The immune system ordinarily generates interferons in response to a virus. Clinical trials proved that giving the MS patient an interferon modulates the way the immune system functions. As a result, it reduced inflammatory MS activity in treated patients by about 30 percent.

In 1996 glatiramer acetate, the first non–interferon MS drug, was released. This medicine is a combination of four amino acids originally designed to look like myelin to the immune system. The development of this drug grew out of work done in 1970 in which researchers discovered that this combination of amino acids cured EAE. Like the interferon drugs, this drug resulted in a reduction in inflammatory MS activity of about 30 percent.

In 1999 there was development of a drug for worsening multiple sclerosis. This drug, mitoxantrone, is a strong immune suppressant still used today, though it has significant side effects (Martinelli et al. 2009).

In a few short years MS patients had come from having no pharmaceutical options to having several. It was widely anticipated that the secondary progressive forms of the disease and later disability would be greatly reduced through successful control of inflammatory relapses due to pharmaceutical innovation, though this has not actually materialized (Pittock et al. 2006; Ebers et al. 2010).

Targeted Immune Suppression

In 2004 the first of a new class of drugs called monoclonal antibodies were released. Natalizumab stops immune cells from leaving the bloodstream and therefore stops most immune system activity in the brain. Unfortunately, this drug sometimes causes opportunistic infections such as progressive multifocal leukoencephalopathy (PML), so it is not used as a first-line drug and must be monitored closely (Berger and Houff 2009). It has an advantage; MRI shows that it results in far less inflammatory activity than previous MS drugs.

People who believe autoimmune activity causes MS view targeted immune approaches like natalizumab as the future of drug therapy. They hope that with further research these kinds of pharmaceuticals can be refined so that the MS patient's precise autoimmune cell can be selectively inactivated, leaving the rest of the immune system intact and functioning normally.

By the end of the 1990s, many experts believed that MS would be a manageable disease if the immune system could be controlled. Today this conviction has grown stronger among the mainstream neurological community.

MS patients have gone from being treated by myth to being persons whose modern care is seen as an example of what is possible with dedication to the evidence-based scientific process. This evidence base gives modern-day physicians scientific assurance about the therapies that they prescribe. There is a sense of pride and anticipation regarding therapies in the research pipeline and a belief that the new therapies will continue to evolve toward a more targeted approach with fewer side effects, as well as a conviction that this direction of research is the correct one.

Understanding the evolution from a position of utter helplessness to one of scientific confidence is important in understanding the professional attitudes of contemporary physicians. However, the current hypotheses are not representative of the whole picture.

Discovery of venous malformations in patients with MS shows there is still more to learn. In the next section information from epidemiological research on MS will be evaluated with a focus on how venous research may be part of that picture.

Findings from Epidemiology

Epidemiology is a word that means the study of a disease from the big-picture view — the people with the disease and the context in which they live from a population perspective.

It is a logic-based science. If all people living next to a lake get ill, one suspects the lake, not genetics. A certain amount of supposition goes into epidemiology because to be meaningful the facts invite some kind of hypothesis to account for what is seen. If it turned out that all people next to that lake were descendants of one person, the answer might lie in genetics after all, so the most obvious answer may not be the correct one. Researchers must always do more studies to confirm the hypothesis suggested by epidemiological findings.

Latitude Gradient and Risk of MS

People who live farther from the equator have higher rates of multiple sclerosis. Individuals living north of the 40th latitude are more likely to have multiple sclerosis. The incidence is a mirror image in the southern hemisphere; individuals who live further south have a higher incidence of MS (Murrell et al. 1991).

Additionally, if a person moves from an area with a low risk of MS to one of high risk before the age of 15, they will acquire the risk of getting MS that matches the new area. If they move after the age of 15, then they will have the MS risk of the place lived in before. Once people reach 15 the risk level seems to be established.

MS experts believe that the difference in risk for northern and southern locations has to do with exposure to sunlight and vitamin D. The epidemiology maps show such a striking increase in these areas, it is easy to speculate that vitamin D plays a role in MS.

Epidemiology research also shows that MS patients as a population tend to have lower serum vitamin D levels than normal controls, and in a large study it was shown that women who use vitamin D supplements had a 40 percent lower risk of MS later in life (Munger et al. 2004). In some way vitamin D must play a role in MS causation.

Some people assume that low vitamin D levels affirm the autoimmune hypothesis because vitamin D modulates the function of the immune system, but there is no evidence that low vitamin D levels could cause people's immune systems to convert to autoimmunity (Chaudhuri 2004); other autoimmune diseases do not have this feature. The scientific fact is that the latitude gradient of MS incidence is unexplained.

The venous model of MS causation does not explain the latitude gradient either. At first glance, it is hard to understand how living in the north would cause an individual's veins to have malformations that would block blood flow. However, vitamin D plays a role in the development of blood vessels and how they function (Sugden et al. 2008; Mitsuhashi et al. 1991; see also Wautier et al. 1996).

Correlation between the latitude lived in specifically before the age of 15 and the risk of MS suggests a developmental issue. Researchers need to investigate the role of vitamin D in the development of the venous system; venous tissue removed from patients with MS shows a congenital (from birth) and developmental origin (Lee et al. 2009).

A study on genetics in 15 people with both CCSVI and MS shows an association between copy number variations in a specific region of the HLA and venous malformations. This area of the genome is associated with the immune system, but the authors cite other work that suggests it also influences angiogenesis (blood vessel creation) (Ferlini et al. 2010).

Infectious Agents: Bacteria and Viruses

Epidemiologic studies show that MS can appear for the first time in a population after exposure to a group of people who come from a high-risk area. This happened in the Faroe Islands after British occupation during World War II.

No Faroese person had ever suffered from a disease that resembled MS prior to British occupation. After the occupation, cases of MS began to develop (Kurtzke and Hyllestad 1979). There were 25 cases diagnosed between 1944 and 1960, showing a striking outbreak. This was speculatively thought to be due to an unidentified bacteria or virus imported with the British, which somehow triggered MS some years later (Kurtzke and Heltberg 2001).

Other recent research has investigated the idea that bacteria or viruses could cause MS as well. Chlamydia pneumoniae (CPn) is a bacterium that causes community-acquired pneumonia. This particular bacterium has unusual survival skills and can live for long periods in a hibernating (latent) state inside the cells of the infected individual.

Research using newer techniques has detected the genetic fingerprint of CPn in the cerebrospinal fluid of people with MS (Fainardi et al. 2009). CPn is also a gram-negative bacterium that produces lipopolysaccharide (LPS). LPS can damage oligodendrocytes (Yao et al. 2010).

A causative association between CPn and MS has not been widely accepted. Some have questioned the research and have published counter-studies arguing against the hypothesis that CPn is causative for MS (Tsai and Gilden 2001).

Others have proposed that CPn is not causative but acts as a co-factor, causing changes that worsen the disease (Fainardi et al. 2008). Yet others suggest it is causative for MS in at least a subset of patients (Stratton and Wheldon 2007). As a result of studies such as these, it is widely understood that there seems to be some scientific evidence of CPn playing a role in MS, but the part this bacterium plays in the development of MS is unclear.

The Epstein Barr virus (EBV) has also repeatedly been associated with MS. The body of evidence showing an association between EBV and MS includes a number of scientific conclusions similar to those that comprise the CPn debate. One recent paper (Pohl et al. 2010) suggests that there is a general immune response to viral peptides in the brains of MS patients but that this is not specific to EBV; the authors show that other viruses are represented in the cerebrospinal fluid as well. The Pohl study suggests that the viral peptides are just an artifact of immune activity rather than evidence of current active infections. In other words, the immune system is active in the brain and on surveillance so the fingerprint of old infections is detectable. The autoimmune model of MS accepts these infectious agents as a theoretical co-factor in the triggering of autoimmunity. The suggestion is that these are not active infections but instead old foes that triggered autoimmune activation.

On the other hand, some people believe active infections are the reason for immune system activity in the MS brain. In this scenario, the solution would be to use medicines that would rid the brain of these infections, such as antibiotics or antiviral drugs.

It is discouraging to realize these questions regarding whether bacteria or viruses trigger MS have been in this state of scientific debate since Pierre Marie first postulated it in 1884. It is still true that nothing is conclusive.

The venous model may be associated with bacteria or viruses in several ways. CPn is a vascular bacterium and strongly associated with atherosclerosis (Gutiérrez et al. 2001). It could possibly play a role in the development of blockages in the veins.

Bacteria and viruses are also more likely to exist in areas impacted by venous insufficiency (Alguire and Mathes 2007). They can cause active or latent infections in the tissue because the tissue has poor blood flow and is unhealthy. For example, CPn has been detected in venous ulcers, which are lesions in the lower leg, caused by venous insufficiency (King et al. 2001).

The Natural Course of MS

MS has been studied for a long time. On a population level the typical disease progression expected in a person with MS is known, although no individual case is strictly average.

Researchers use the EDSS scale to measure the average rate of progression in MS patients. Recall that the EDSS quantifies MS with assigned values of 0–10. The following table is adapted from FDA materials.

EDSS 1   No disability but minimal signs of neurological problems in one system.

EDSS 2   Minimal disability in one functional system.

EDSS 3   Moderate disability in one functional system or mild disability in 3 systems. This person is still ambulatory without a cane or assistive device.

EDSS 4   This person is fully ambulatory without aid and up 12 hours a day despite relatively severe disability, but is able to walk 500 meters without aid or rest.

EDSS 5   This person is able to walk 200 meters without aid or rest. Disability restricts daily activity and lifestyle may require modifications.

EDSS 6   This person uses a cane, crutch or brace at all times and can walk 100 meters with or without resting.

EDSS 7   This person can walk no more than 5 meters and depends on a wheelchair; however, they transfer alone and can wheel themselves, staying up and active 12 hours a day.

EDSS 8   This person is restricted to bed but is still able to use their arms for some self-care functions and able to communicate.

EDSS 9   This person is restricted to bed.

EDSS 10 Death due to MS.

Adapted from FDA.gov; descriptions of half-steps such as 1.5, 2.5, etc., left out.

A study published in 2006 on progression, provocatively titled "Disability Progression Is Slower in MS than Previously Reported," evaluated MS patients to see when, on average, they reached disability touch-points of EDSS 3, 6 and 8. The information for this study came from a large database in British Columbia that included a whopping 22,728 patient years and a group of patients 2,837 strong. Patients evaluated for this study had to have been diagnosed prior to 1988, so available data covered a minimum of 15 years (Tremlett et al. 2006).

This study found that on average people with MS do not reach EDSS 6 until 27.9 years after initial symptoms emerge. At the 15-year mark, only 21 percent of patients needed a cane. The researchers determined that at the 40-year mark 31 percent of study participants were still walking unassisted. In this clinic, people were evaluated an average of every 1.1 years, so there was ample data to pinpoint changes in function. Only 15.5 percent of these patients took a disease-modifying drug and these patients showed a slightly more rapid progression; the authors attributed this to the idea that people who took the drugs were the people who were progressing (Tremlett et al. 2006).

According to another study, MS patients typically become progressive at 39 years of age. This research noted that an RRMS patient will become secondary progressive at about that age, and PPMS patients are diagnosed at about that age. In the view of these researchers, times to reach disability milestones happen on a preset schedule tied to age and relapses do not influence this schedule (Confavreux and Vukusic 2006).

Another population-based study looked for markers that would identify the patients with benign disease. Benign MS is defined as a person who has an EDSS of 2 or less 10 years after diagnosis. Such a person has a 93 percent chance of remaining stable over the next 10 years. This study established the portion of the population with benign disease as a significantly large 17 percent (Pittock et al. 2004).

These population-based studies on the natural history of MS highlight the fact that, on average, MS is a slow-moving disease and a significant subset of people with MS have benign disease.

This explains why it is so difficult to investigate new pharmaceuticals: the time frame that is reasonable for a clinical trial is not long enough to learn what impact the drug has on progressive illness. Additionally, progression may not be obvious in a population of people with MS for many years if people are treated at a young age or early in the disease simply because it is too soon for progression to be seen.

It is easy to see why pharmaceutical researchers have a difficult time understanding how a trial drug impacts progression in studies that are usually 2 years long. A recent controversy highlights this issue.

The National Health Service (NHS) and Drug Data

The national healthcare system in the United Kingdom, the NHS, made a special arrangement with each of the makers of the first-tier drugs — the interferons and glatiramer acetate. When the pharmaceutical companies introduced these drugs, the NHS had originally determined that the clinical trials had too little evidence to show that they slowed the actual disease process to warrant the use of the drugs. In order to tap into the UK market for MS drugs, the pharmaceutical manufacturers agreed that the drugs would be available under a special arrangement called the "risk-sharing scheme." UK MS patients would be allowed to have the drugs and physicians would monitor these patients over time. The NHS would tie compensation for the companies to how much healthier treated patients were than untreated people (Raferty 2010).

Unfortunately, the review of patient progress over time showed that patients treated with these drugs did worse than predicted by the company's clinical research studies. Unexpectedly, the treated people also seemed to progress faster than the untreated historical comparison group (Boggild et al. 2009). The number of patients evaluated was over 5,500, which makes the findings significant. A quote from the paper follows:

> In the primary per protocol analysis, progression in disability was worse than that predicted and worse than that in the untreated comparator dataset ("deviation score" of 113%; excess in mean disability status scale 0.28). In sensitivity analyses, however, the deviation score varied from -72% (using raw baseline disability status scale scores, rather than applying a "no improvement" algorithm) to 156% (imputing missing data for year two from progression rates for year one) [Boggild et al. 2009].

The problems with the statistics led the authors to conclude that it was too soon to make firm statements about the effectiveness of these drugs. They recommended that the NHS should continue to monitor these patients over time for conclusive results.

The cautious course of action is not entirely about the data. It has some roots in the politics of the medical dynamic. Realistically, the idea of summarily taking all the people in the NHS off these drugs is unconscionable. The NHS could only undertake such a radical action if it could be proven that this outcome, which is substantially different from previous research, is accurate. The problems with data make that questionable.

This is a real-life example of the difficulty in trying to decide in a short study whether a drug impacts progression or not, and how epidemiology may shed light on the ways pharmaceuticals affect real people. Another issue that population studies can evaluate this way is the relative contribution of relapses and inflammatory activity to eventual disability in MS patients.

Inflammation, Degeneration, Atrophy and Disability

Relapses in patients with MS naturally diminish in number as time goes by even without any treatment. It is also well known that disability and degenerative changes in the brain increase over time. Disability is highly correlated with atrophy in the brain and is thought to be due to loss of axons (Miller et al. 2002).

Functional losses that occur during relapses are caused by demyelination and inflammation. These usually remit after the relapse is over. Patients who are still relapsing and remitting tend to have swings, up and down, in the EDSS numbers due to relapse impact on EDSS scale (Coyle 2006). On the other hand, degeneration and atrophy do not remit. Changes in EDSS caused by degeneration are permanent. These are progressive losses of nerves themselves, not just dysfunction of nerves. It is the second of these phenomena that is the cause of progression and permanent disability.

The widely held view is that inflammatory relapses somehow cause later degeneration, atrophy and progressive disability; the theory is that repeated bouts of inflammation eventually damage the nerve over time.

However, there is research that seems to suggest the "inflammation first" hypothesis may be missing something. The following comment was made in a paper evaluating nerve damage and inflammation in MS patients:

> No correlation was found between whole brain NAA concentrations and lesion volumes. Widespread axonal pathology, largely independent of MRI-visible inflammation and too extensive to be completely reversible, occurs in patients even at the earliest clinical stage of multiple sclerosis. This finding lessens the validity of the current concept that the axonal pathology of multiple sclerosis is the end-stage result of repeated inflammatory events, and argues strongly in favour of early neuroprotective intervention [Filippi et al. 2003].

The amino acid compound n-acetyl aspartate (NAA) is a naturally occurring metabolite that is reduced when there is nerve damage. The researchers are saying that the MS brain, even early in the disease with low lesion loads, has been shown to have very reduced NAA levels and widespread damage to axons independent of inflammatory lesions that were visible on MRI (Filippi et al. 2003). This suggests the lowered NAA, an early sign of degeneration, precedes inflammatory lesions.

Another research group suggests that axonal loss is not related to MS plaques (lesions): "Unexpectedly, after adjusting for sex, age and duration of disease, correlations between total plaque load and axonal loss in both the corticospinal tract and sensory tracts were weak or absent at each level investigated. Since there was little correlation between plaque load and axonal loss, the possibility that demyelination is not the primary determinant of spinal cord axonal loss warrants consideration" (Deluca et al. 2006).

Another research team argues against the idea that inflammation is the cause of much later degenerative changes, pointing out that the patient who presents with optic neuritis does not experience onset of secondary progression with blindness. They claim this disputes the *compartmentalization* argument for early inflammation causing late degeneration (Scalfari et al. 2010). Compartmentalization is the theory that inflammation leaves degenerative factors behind that cause damage much later, which some have proposed could be the cause of late degeneration in the MS brain.

Recent research looking at iron deposits as a marker for degeneration in 970 patients has shown that in people with MS iron loads increase over time. When nerves die, they leave iron behind. However, in some patients with low lesion loads, there was *greater* iron content than in another group with high lesion loads. The authors argue that this supports the idea that MS is primarily degenerative (Burgetova et al. 2010). These papers above indicate a possibility that axonal loss is the primary issue in MS, meaning degeneration exists prior to and independent of inflammation.

It also appears that inflammatory lesions may not cause disability and progression. One group mentions that as time goes on the dissociation between inflammation and disability becomes more apparent (Kremenchutzky et al. 2006). They comment that current drugs suppress inflammation effectively and should be reducing progressive disability if inflammation is the cause of progressive illness; they argue this is not materializing.

Tsutsui and Stys (2009) make this comment in their paper: "Curiously, and perhaps counterintuitive to the notion of inflammation as a major driver of progressive disability, relapses do not significantly influence later progression."

Another team of researchers made this comment:

> All these observations give support to the fact that relapses do not essentially influence irreversible disability in the long term in MS ... [and] suggests MS is as much neurodegenerative as inflammatory, and should cause the modification of disease-modifying therapeutic strategies by focusing on the protection and repair of the nervous system and not only on the control of inflammation [Confavreux and Vukusic 2006a].

In 2010 a large population-based study evaluating 806 patients' progression (28,000 patient years) confirmed the earlier authors' thoughts on these points, adding that relapses in the first two years have a modest predictive value for eventual disability; if there were more than 3 relapses, then the person had an increased chance of faster progression. However, relapses after the second year had an inverse relationship to disability; in other words, relapses in later years suggested slower progression. The authors conclude,

"These data should further discourage any direct causal relationship between clinical attack numbers and disability accumulation" (Scalfari et al. 2010).

Altogether, these papers suggest that progressive disease and disability are not a direct consequence of inflammation. Some people think the reason this correlation is not clear is because the immune system suppression simply has not been complete enough. The next section discusses stronger immune system suppression.

Effectiveness of Autologous Stem Cell Transplants

Some people suggest that this lack of a clear connection between inflammation and disability is due to the fact that MS patients need stronger suppression of the immune system. Autologous stem cell transplant (ASCT) is the extreme form of immune system suppression because it removes the current immune system completely, then replaces it with a new one. Theoretically, this reboot of immune function will end autoimmune attacks.

In this radical therapy, a patient is administered some version of strong chemotherapy, and sometimes radiation as well, to completely remove their immune system. The patient is at grave risk during the phase where the immune system is gone; they must be in the hospital in protective isolation. The patient then receives stem cells harvested from their body before the procedure to rebuild a new, healthy immune system. The new system is completely naïve and has no memory of bacteria, viruses or other foreign antigens it learned to attack before; the person who undergoes ASCT with chemotherapy to remove the old immune system must be re-immunized with what are commonly referred to as baby shots. Theoretically, this newly minted immune system will "forget" to attack the brain, bringing an end to MS.

This approach should work well to repair autoimmunity, yet some research indicates it does not appear to stop degeneration in MS. In one study, 4 autopsy samples from people who had died after a stem cell transplant for MS showed almost a complete absence of inflammatory cells. However, these patients had evidence of ongoing axonal damage, indicating that "even though inflammation had been abolished, neurodegeneration was still proceeding in the brains of these patients and thus that neurodegeneration is not a consequence, at least in the short term, of inflammation" (Bruck 2005).

In a study on ASCT that compared several diseases the patients with the autoimmune diseases lupus and juvenile arthritis had their diseases arrested, but unfortunately MS patients did not fare well; the procedure only stopped progression in a minority of multiple sclerosis patients (Brinkman et al. 2007). Other research teams also document progression after ASCT, though the disease stabilized in the majority for three to five years before progressing again (Krasulova et al. 2010; Farge et al. 2010).

Another research group also argues ASCT fails to stop damage in the MS brain. Researchers documented degeneration in absence of inflammatory cells when looking at 5 autopsy samples from people who died after ASCT.

> The present results indicate that ongoing demyelination and axonal degeneration exist despite pronounced immunosuppression. Our data parallel results from some of the clinical phase I/II studies showing continued clinical disease progression in multiple sclerosis patients with high expanded disability system scores despite autologous stem cell transplantation [Metz et al. 2007].

A different research team argued that the conclusions drawn by the Metz research team were incomplete. They suggest the problem could be that patients were too far progressed with too many degenerative changes in the brain to be helped by suppressing their immune function (Nash et al. 2008). Others have also argued that there is a "window of therapeutic opportunity" and postulate that suppression of inflammation could only prevent disability if done very early in the disease (Coles et al. 2009).

However, aggressive suppression of immune system function is inherently dangerous; working immune systems are necessary for health. Though treatment is getting safer, occasionally patients die from ASCT (Rogojan and Frederiksen 2009). As a result, most physicians do not consider something like ASCT unless the patient progresses while taking safer therapies or the patient has malignant MS (unusually rapid decline to disability). This does appear to be a very important saving strategy for patients with malignant MS; according to one research team, it "is not a treatment for the general MS population but only for selected cases that do not respond to standard therapy" (Fassas and Mancardi 2008). Of course, this means MS patients are considered for these aggressive therapies after they have progressed, bringing the argument back to the idea that, if used after people have progressed, it could theoretically be too late to stop degeneration.

One problem preventing resolution of the degeneration versus inflammation debate is no one has discovered any verifiable cause for degeneration that predates inflammation. MS is always discovered when inflammation is present; it is inflammation that is seen on MRI in lesions, inflammation that causes relapses, and inflammation that is proven to be impacted with all of the MS drugs. Is it possible that researchers have been distracted by inflammation, as if inflammation is multiple sclerosis when in fact it's primarily degenerative, with inflammation secondary?

As discussed earlier, it appears that inflammation is not consistently correlated with disability or degeneration, which seem to progress in spite of controlling inflammation. Even ASCT, which completely replaces the immune system, eventually allows progression in the majority of patients. The venous model may possibly offer a solution to this conundrum.

Venous malformations could theoretically be the root cause of MS degeneration and inflammation alike. Venous insufficiency in the leg causes aggressive inflammation and degeneration of tissue in the lower leg (see chapter 4).

Speculatively, if venous insufficiency damages MS brains in some way similar to what occurs in legs with venous insufficiency, this could account for the fact that inflammation can easily be reduced with today's standard MS therapies but degeneration and progression slowly continue. Theoretically, the result could be ongoing damage without inflammation if the drug controls inflammation but venous problems remain.

The question of whether MS is primarily inflammatory or primarily degenerative needs an answer before a true cure can be discovered. Until that happens, treating inflammation may or may not have a long-term impact on the disease

Heterogeneity

It is widely accepted that MS is a heterogeneous disease, meaning it is a variable illness with possibly more than one causative agent, thus accounting for the various symptoms. There may be subtypes or variants of MS. Research and its ongoing lack of conclusiveness are thought to be due to this heterogeneity. For example, perhaps only some people have autoimmune MS. Perhaps another subset has been infected with one of the infectious agents discussed earlier.

MS clearly presents in a heterogeneous way with the various forms of RRMS, SPMS and PPMS. The timetable is also unique for individuals and largely unpredictable even within these classifications. Some patients seem to do well on drug A, while others seem to do better on drug B; this seems to further confirm the idea of heterogeneity.

The NMSS decided to fund a major project to evaluate lesions on a microscopic level to see if there were any differences between patients. The direction of this research was suggested by work indicating there may be several lesion types. The hope was that they would discover the difference between subtypes of MS at this level, resulting in a major breakthrough.

Prominent researchers in the field of MS from all over the world were recruited to be part of this lesion project. Claudia Lucchinetti, MD, from the Mayo Clinic was the project leader. The NMSS website states the project has amassed an extensive database over 10 years of study. Autopsy and biopsy provided the tissue samples for the researchers. They have identified four lesion types.

According to the research team, an individual with MS has only one of the four lesion types and all of that person's lesions are of that type. Lesion types I and II appear to have characteristics similar to encephalomyelitis. The type II lesion differs from type I in that it shows immunoglobins and complement, and this suggests a type of immune system cell called a B cell is involved in that lesion type. Types III and IV show more prominent oligodendrocyte damage and are thought to be more similar to damage caused by toxic or viral triggers (Lucchinetti et al. 2000). More research needs to be done to understand what these differences may mean for MS patients.

The work by this team of researchers has been widely accepted and appreciated. It suggests that patients with treatment failures are simply not the type of MS to do well on that particular therapy.

The hope is that eventually therapy can be tailored to match the type of lesion in an individual. For example, the type II lesions showed B cell involvement. Such a person would possibly do better on a drug that reduces B cells. Many people in the MS community hailed this work with a sense of relief that MS research finally had an explanation for the significant number of people who fail standard therapies.

However, MS research is often back and forth. This question regarding the heterogeneity of lesions is no exception to that rule. Others have tried to replicate the original group's findings and have not seen the same thing. Rather, homogeneity (sameness) has been noted.

> INTERPRETATION: The immunopathological appearance of active demyelinating lesions in established MS is uniform. Initial heterogeneity of demyelinating lesions in the earliest phase of MS lesion formation may disappear over time as different pathways converge in one general mechanism of demyelination. Consistent presence of complement, antibodies, and Fcgamma receptors in phagocytic macrophages suggests that antibody- and complement-mediated myelin phagocytosis is the dominant mechanism of demyelination in established MS [Breij et al. 2008].

This means that when this group assessed active lesions they saw the same kind of immune cells in all the lesions of persons with established MS. This suggests it is not likely that people need widely different therapies. They propose that the reason they saw one type when the lesion project saw four is that perhaps four types of early lesions evolve into the single pattern this group saw. Another researcher submitted a positive comment supporting the conclusions drawn by the Breij research (Raine 2008).

This is not the only team to offer an opinion supporting homogenous lesions. Barnett and colleagues (2006) offer this observation:

> The presence of such lesions in patients with a spectrum of pathological changes in nearby or distant active phagocytic plaques suggests that pathological heterogeneity in MS is largely due to evolution of lesional pathology, rather than pathogenic heterogeneity.

This is saying that, in their opinion, the heterogeneity seen in the lesion project was due to the evolution of the lesion, not differences in the basic disease. The biopsy samples used in the lesion project represent a select group of atypical patients who are having trouble being diagnosed, not typical MS patients.

Another group of researchers also noted homogeneity. They mention lesion location seems to determine whether complement is in the lesion or not: "In conclusion, the role of complement in MS pathogenesis seems lesion location-dependent" (Brink et al. 2005).

In an earlier work Barnett and Prineas documented that oligodendrocytes died prior to immune activation in MS patients. This phenomenon was seen in newly forming lesions in autopsy samples of all patients, which suggests homogeneity in the initial event (Barnett and Prineas 2004).

Another researcher offered this comment regarding the lesion project and its effort to discover different lesion types:

> Although this approach has merit, concern has been expressed regarding the details of the cases on which it is based and whether the central nervous system-biopsy specimens examined came from patients with typical multiple sclerosis. Furthermore, Barnett and Prineas have recently demonstrated that lesions from a given patient can, in fact, contain features of more than one category of lesions. This important observation underscores the fact that the development of a cogent and accurate lesion-classification scheme remains a work in progress [Frohman et al. 2006].

It is important to keep in mind that the heterogeneity of MS lesions remains an unproven hypothesis proposed by a single group of researchers. Efforts to reproduce this study have not yielded the same results and other questions have been raised.

Plain-Language Summary and Comment

The fact that MS lesions occur on venules of a certain size has been known since the 1800s. Attempts to investigate venous causation of MS in the 1950s failed because diagnostic technology was not available. Instead, crude approaches limited to simple anticoagulation, temporary vasodilation, and wacky "circulation stimulators" were used, then rejected as useless. Meanwhile, the immune model came to be viewed as the best hypothesis for MS causation because research findings repeatedly uncovered connections between MS lesions and the immune system. EAE provided a way to do controlled experiments with reliable scientific findings on immune system activity in brains of mice.

As research developed data over the years, it became clear that inflammation is the cause of relapses through demyelination and immune activity in the brain; remyelination and reduction of inflammation results in a return of function and remission. RRMS causes swings up and down in EDSS scores.

Today's standard therapies reduce this inflammatory activity. Conversely, the progressive phase of the disease is caused by degeneration and loss of nerves themselves, and increasingly researchers are identifying degeneration as a separate problem and not simply a result of inflammation that occurred earlier. Stem cell transplants are the most radical and aggressive version of immune system suppression, yet even this approach seems to allow continued degenerative loss of nerves.

This has implications for the potential of therapies that control inflammation to actually control the disease. Some have argued that progressive nerve degeneration is the more important aspect of multiple sclerosis and research should evolve toward developing strategies that affect this part of the disease rather than focusing entirely on inflammatory relapses.

However, the problem preventing this shift is that it is extremely difficult to evaluate the impact pharmaceuticals have on the progressive phase of the disease. Population studies have revealed why this is difficult. People seem to become progressive at about the age of 39. It also seems to take many years after initial symptoms before actual progression caused by degenerative changes becomes obvious in most people, and 17 percent of people with MS have benign disease, which means that a significant portion of any group of tested individuals should do very well even on an ineffective therapy. These facts, taken together, make it very difficult to determine if a pharmaceutical impacts the progressive phase of the disease, although it is not difficult to prove these drugs reduce the inflammatory relapses and stabilize EDSS scores, which is a reasonable therapeutic goal.

MS research has evolved in a direction that can be termed reductionist, going from looking at the MS patient as a whole being of interacting systems to looking through the microscope at the cells present in the lesion. The MS lesion project, with its unreplicated findings, is a good example of this direction of research and reveals the belief held by most that MS is exclusively an immunological problem. The people who decided that the lesion project would be the major focus of research assumed from the outset that the cause of this illness is discernable at the microscopic level, which may not be the case and reveals a predetermined bias toward the cause of MS. Immune system activity caused by venous insufficiency may look like autoimmune activity at this microscopic level (see chapter 4). It is also possible that venous insufficiency triggers autoimmune activity. Seen from this point of view, research investigating the vascular connection to MS is all the more urgent.

However, there is a vast database about the immune system activation in MS. Even if MS was a venous disease, this immune-focused research is still very pertinent to the lesion pathology. The immune system damages the brain of an MS patient and decades of research show just how extensive that damage is. Obviously, if MS is a primary venous pathology, then this includes extensive immune system involvement as a secondary part of the disease process. An overview of the immune system and how it behaves in MS is reviewed in the next chapter.

3

The Immune System
and Autoimmunity in MS

A backbone is better than a wishbone — posted on TIMS

Immune system activity is present in MS lesions. It also causes much of the damage to the MS brain tissue. Research on how the immune system impacts MS is still of critical interest, even in the venous model. In fact, some immune system research supports the possibility that venous insufficiency plays a role in MS.

The immune system is explained in the first part of this chapter. The autoimmune model is then explored with that background. This is followed by research that suggests MS may *not* be autoimmune.

The first part of this chapter is the most complicated information in this book. The immune system is extremely complex and not easily remembered without extensive study; use this chapter as a primer for reference as you read later chapters.

The Immune System

The body is in a constant state of cellular life and death. The immune system removes individual cells when they reach the end of their natural life cycle so new cells can take their place. This keeps the body healthy and constantly renewed.

Tumor cells are removed as part of normal immune system activity. The immune system identifies these cells and destroys them. Effective immune system function is important to remaining cancer-free (Berger and Houff 2009).

The immune system is also responsible for killing and/or removing toxins, bacteria, parasites and viruses; antigens on each cell's surface identify these organisms. Antigens are an important signal to the immune system because they identify a cell as being part of the self, or, conversely, as a "foreign" cell to attack.

The immune system uses white blood cells — including T cells and B cells (lymphocytes), macrophages, monocytes and neutrophils, complement, cytokines, interleukins, interferons and adhesion molecules — to keep the body under constant immune surveillance. Understanding the immune system makes understanding MS easier even if there is a venous component. Antigens are a good place to start.

Antigens

Antigens are protein and carbohydrate molecules that exist on the outside of cells. These molecules identify the cell to the immune system. The immune system has this ability to "read" antigens so it can differentiate self cells from foreign ones. Think of antigens as nametags, such as "foreign-bacteria" or "self-heart," that are worn on the outside of the cell in a special receptor. These molecules vary from species to species and from individual to individual. Self antigens are readily tolerated by the immune system while foreign antigens are aggressively attacked by immune cells.

The body usually successfully differentiates self antigens from foreign antigens. Autoimmunity occurs when the immune system attacks the cells of the self as if they were foreign.

The complex interplay of immune system factors that results in healthy immunity takes many different cellular components to reach that goal. Antigens are the key to correct identification for all the components.

Innate or Non-Specific Immunity

Every human being is born with the ability to protect themselves from bacteria and viruses even without having specific antibodies against them. This is called *innate* immunity.

An important feature of innate immunity is *phagocytes*, which are white blood cells that eat bacteria and viruses as well as scavenge in the body to remove dead tissue. The term *phagocytosing a cell* means to absorb and digest it. Macrophages are sometimes referred to as *big eaters*.

Phagocytes are able to move to an area where there is a damaged cell. The damaged cell emits a *chemo-attractant*, a chemical signal, that attracts immune system cells to the area.

Once a phagocyte ingests a foreign bacteria, virus or cell, it *presents the antigen* to the rest of the immune system by putting it in a special receptor on its surface. Think of this as if the phagocyte has taken the nametag from the invader and put it in the receptor so the other immune system cells will recognize it and attack it. Antigen presenting is a critical step in the immune cascade because it starts the process that results in a specific, targeted immune response, such as production of antibodies and activation of T cells.

Specific Immunity Targeting Specific Antigens

Non-specific immunity, described above, protects people from infectious agents before a targeted response can begin. "Specific immunity" is how the body targets individual foreign cells in a precise attack.

Specific immunity has two separate arms that work together to accomplish the goal of targeting and removing foreign invaders. Humoral immunity and cellular immunity will be discussed separately.

HUMORAL IMMUNITY: B CELLS AND ANTIBODY PRODUCTION • Humoral immunity is immune activity that is initiated by a type of lymphocyte known as a B cell, which that circulates in body fluids, such as blood and lymph. Lymphocytes are also referred to as white blood cells.

On the surface of every B cell are immunoglobins, which will bind to foreign antigens offered on antigen-presenting cells — for example, the phagocyte mentioned earlier. The B cell absorbs the antigen, disassembles it, then makes antibodies for that specific antigen. It also divides and multiplies, passing this new information about the antigen to its clones to increase the immune response.

The B cells release antibodies into the circulatory system, allowing them to move freely throughout the body. These antibodies are immunoglobins. The most common immunoglobins are immunoglobin G (IgG) and immunoglobin M (IgM). B cells make IgM antibodies plentifully in a first encounter with a foreign antigen; repeat encounters with the antigen result in IgG antibodies. The fact that there are IgG oligoclonal bands in MS indicates B cell activity in the brains of MS patients.

When antibodies encounter the target antigen on the cell surface of a foreign invader somewhere in the body, they will bind to that antigen, thus "marking" that cell for destruction by other cells of the immune system, such as the phagocytes mentioned earlier or complement. Antibodies can also neutralize some toxins on their own.

The B cells also maintain *memory*; by regularly making a few cells that recognize that antigen, the immune system will recognize it if encountered later in life — this is how vaccination works. The B cells will be able to activate

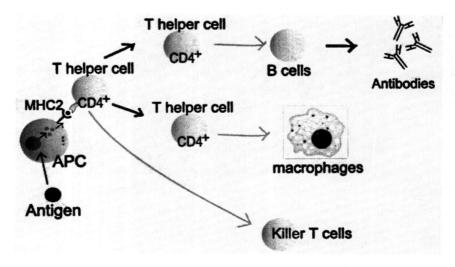

This schematic representation shows the sequence of events that results in a targeted immune system response. The antigen is absorbed by an antigen-presenting cell (APC). The APC puts the nametag part of the cell in its MHC II receptor. The CD4 cells co-stimulate other processes so that the B cells can make antibodies that will attack the antigen, macrophages can seek out and eat the antigen, and cytotoxic killer cells can destroy cells bearing that antigen.

and make antibodies for that antigen very quickly if it is ever detected in the body again, destroying it before it can replicate and make the person ill. This ability to recognize and attack formerly encountered antigens usually lasts for the life of the individual.

Complement has the ability to destroy other cells if activated. A cell with an antibody attached is one way to activate complement. It is also capable of working on its own in certain circumstances. Complement is an enzymatic protein that dissolves other cells; phagocytes then eat/remove the debris.

The complement system can also be involved in removal of dead cells. Cells at the end of their natural life begin to display an altered-self antigen. Think of the nametag in this situation as saying "needing assisted suicide."

Recent research suggests the B cells are part of the immune cell activity seen in the MS brain. Activated complement, oligoclonal bands, and B cells have been detected in MS lesions. These new findings are counter to the common view that MS immune system activity is driven by T cells; understanding about immune system activity in MS is constantly broadening.

T CELLS AND CELLULAR IMMUNITY • Antibody-making B cells are one type of lymphocyte; another type of lymphocyte is the T cell. Like B cells, T cells are made in the bone marrow. However, instead of maturing in the lymph tissue, the T cells mature in the thymus.

T cells are important to targeted immunity. T cells are either CD4 or CD8 phenotype. There are both CD4 and CD8 cells in MS lesions and the animal model of MS mentioned previously, EAE, though the balance is different when comparing MS and EAE.

The CD8 cells produce two types of cells. One type is T suppressor cells, which control the immune reaction through the use of cytokines by suppressing some immune activities.

The other type of CD8 cells are cytotoxic T lymphocytes (CTLs). Antigen-presenting cells, such as phagocytes with the antigen "nametag" in the receptor, activate CTL cells so they will attack a specific foreign antigen. The CTL can destroy the cell showing that antigen. These cells clonally expand themselves (make clones by dividing to increase numbers) when activated. MS lesions have many CD8+ clonally expanded cells in them.

"Cyto" means cell; "cytotoxic" is a descriptive term for what these cells do. The CTL attacks by injecting proteinases and enzymes that break down the structure of the cell, eventually triggering cell death. The debris is removed by a phagocyte. This makes it possible for the immune system to destroy cells that have viruses or bacteria inside of them; this ability is an important part of cellular immunity.

The CD4 cells are commonly called T helper (TH) lymphocytes. These cells direct and manage other immune processes to control immune function. The helpers can be activated in a TH1 or TH2 pattern. The TH1 is a type of response typically activated for infections and is marked by inflammation. TH2 reactions are more often associated with hypersensitivity or allergic types of responses.

The helper cells also co-stimulate other immune processes — for example, activation of B cells. They do this by activating yet another type of molecule: cytokines. The type and combination of cytokines activated differs in TH1 and TH2 responses. MS appears to be a TH1 type of immune response.

The cytokines that the TH cells co-stimulate are able to activate or block the function of other immune cells. Cytokines bring about a milder immune response in certain combinations and a very strong immune response in others. Cytokines are essentially the traffic cops of the immune system, controlling the activities of the numerous members of the immune cascade.

CYTOKINES • Cytokines include many interleukins, interferons, tumor necrosis factors, colony stimulating factors, transforming growth factors, and chemokines. These chemical messengers regulate other immune activities. Some of these cytokines are mutually exclusive and in other cases mutually synergistic, and sometimes, depending on a third cytokine, they might even be both!

Inflammation is a consequence of cytokine activity. Inflammation is technically the migration of plasma (the fluid part of the blood), cytokines, and white blood cells out of circulation and into the tissue. Inflammation *is* immune activity to a great extent.

Adhesion molecules are an example of something that enhances inflammation; they cause the immune system cells to adhere to the blood vessel wall and then to migrate out into the tissue. Cytokines then stimulate the immune system cells to repair the area. This cytokine-mediated immune system activity results in congestion in the local tissue, which is seen as redness and swelling. The MS drug natalizumab reduces adhesion molecule function.

There are also *anti*-inflammatory cytokines and some are activated at the same time as the inflammatory types. Examples of these are interleukin 4 (IL4), IL10, and interferons. These control inflammation. The interferons have been exploited for MS through being made into injectable drugs.

By various methods of checks and balances where some components cause more immune activation and others cause less, the system regulates itself so that there are no out-of-control immune reactions and inflammation.

MHC: ANTIGEN PRESENTING AND RECOGNIZING SELF • Major histocompatibility complex, or MHC, is the grouping of molecules on the outside of cells that identifies them — essentially, the antigen mentioned earlier. In humans this is called human leukocyte antigen, or HLA.

There are two kinds of MHC/HLA. Class I MHC is on all cells of the body and tells the immune system, "I am self." On foreign cells, the MHC identifies the cell as foreign. Class I MHC talks about what is going on inside the cell — what kind of cell it is.

If the cell is a healthy self cell, there will be self antigens in the MHC region. If there is a virus inside, some of the viral peptides will be in the MHC, marking the cell for attack. If the cell is damaged or old, altered peptides will be exposed in the MHC and this will also result in immune attack.

Class II MHC is on the immune cells and is involved with antigen presenting. Phagocytes, B cells and activated T cells all have class II MHC, which is used to present the antigens of something going on *outside* the immune cell presenting it. This antigen presentation is what primes the immune system to attack a certain foreign invader. Here's an example: A phagocyte eats a bacteria. It disassembles the bacteria and presents some of the bacterial cells in its class II MHC so other cells of the immune system, like T cells, are activated against that antigen. Antigens presented in a class II MHC are targeted by the immune system for attack.

The class II MHC matters in MS because about 50 percent of MS patients have a certain genetic type of HLA molecule: HLA DR2 (Modin et al. 2004). Some suggest this is confirmation of autoimmunity, assuming that this type is prone to misdirect immune function because T cells know what to attack and what to ignore based on MHC II activity. But not all people with MS have HLA DR2. And most people with HLA DR2 do not have MS (Murrell et al. 1991).

VACCINES • Vaccines induce an immune response by giving the individual an inactive antigen so that the immune cascade is primed to attack that antigen. Being inactive, the antigen cannot cause the disease itself. It is as if the vaccine is just the "nametag" part of the target cell.

It is possible to use a self antigen to create a vaccine against a self tissue. This is done by taking an antigen from that tissue and altering it so that it will be seen as foreign, often by irradiating it. By this method it is possible to prime the immune system to attack problematic self cells such as tumor cells or autoimmune cells.

This area of research shows promise because it might be possible to alter the immune system in a targeted way. The hope is to find the exact immune system cell that is causing the autoimmunity and knock out only that one cell by teaching the immune system to recognize that cell as foreign. Researchers have not yet discovered such a cell in MS.

Although immune system activity in the central nervous system (CNS) causes damage through inflammation, research is increasingly showing that the immune cells also trigger healing (Rock et al. 2004). Inflammatory immune cells in the CNS appear to be a double-edged sword, both healing and damaging.

Summary of the Healthy Immune System

This limited review of the immune system brings to light important features of the immune system that may play a role in multiple sclerosis. As MS is discussed later in this chapter, this list can serve as a quick reference:

1. Non-specific or innate immunity allows scavenging and attack without programming ahead of time. The phagocytes are important to innate immunity and present antigens to the other cells of the immune system in a type II MHC after identifying a problem cell.
2. *Microglia*, often mentioned in relation to MS, are simply macrophages behind the blood-brain barrier and are the brain's resident immune cells.

3. B cells make antibodies to target foreign cells. Foreign cells are "coated" with antibodies marking them for attack by complement. Phagocytes remove the debris after complement has dissolved the cell.
4. T cells are activated when an antigen is presented in a type II MHC.
5. Helper T cells, CD4+, aid other immune activities by directing cytokines and chemokines, which co-stimulate other immune activities.
6. Cytotoxic T cells, CD8+, can be activated to target a specific antigen. The cytotoxic element breaks down the proteins of the targeted cell with enzymes and proteases. Complement and natural killers function similarly but are not restricted to one antigenic target. All work in slightly different ways under different conditions. Phagocytes scavenge debris after the fact.
7. Inflammation goes hand in hand with immune cell activity. Cytokines control inflammation with both pro-inflammatory and anti-inflammatory types. The balance varies in TH1 and TH2 patterns.
8. HLA is the human MHC and is genetically encoded. It's involved with antigen presenting and discernment between self and non-self.

Immune function usually keeps people healthy by removing foreign invaders and repairing and maintaining the cells. This complex system works surprisingly well, but sometimes there is a mistake in the system. Autoimmunity is such a mistake.

General Description of Autoimmunity

Healthy cells are targeted by the immune system in autoimmunity. Surprisingly, a few autoimmune cells are normal (Schwartz and Kipnis 2002).

Autoimmune cells are present in healthy persons and these cells are part of cellular maintenance. It is not normal for autoimmunity to go beyond normal levels of healing and repair with these self-reactive cells, however. The immune system usually keeps the autoimmune aspect of immune function tightly regulated with cytokines and by triggering the self-reactive cells to die after a short period of time (Yoles et al. 2001). When the natural level of autoimmune function is too high, it becomes an *autoimmune disease.*

Autoimmune disease occurs when healthy cells are attacked beyond the level of normal maintenance and the tissue is actually damaged instead of maintained or repaired.

For the purposes of this book, there are two classes of autoimmune diseases. Classic autoimmune diseases are those diseases where the mechanism of the autoimmunity is clearly understood and research has identified the specific antigen that is being targeted by the immune system. Rheumatic fever is such a disease.

The other type of autoimmune disease is a disease that is thought to be autoimmune but does not have conclusive research proving an autoimmune mechanism. Multiple sclerosis falls into this second category.

Rheumatic Fever

Rheumatic fever is a classic autoimmune disease. What happens in rheumatic fever is a person becomes ill with a certain strain of strep throat and does not get treatment with antibiotics before an aggressive immune system reaction occurs as the body tries to fight off the bacteria.

Unfortunately, in some people the antibodies made to fight off the strep bacteria cross-react with their heart and/or joint tissue, causing damage to the heart and an aggressive inflammatory arthritis. This autoimmune reaction is self-limited; the immune system cells naturally die off and the symptoms of the disease ease away, though the person may have permanent heart and joint damage left over from the ravages of the accidental autoimmune attack. People who have had rheumatic fever will take care for the rest of their lives to avoid such a reaction again by taking antibiotics if they should have a sore throat or dental work, thus preventing the immune system going into overdrive and triggering autoimmunity again.

The thing to note about this is that it does stop; the controlling factors of the immune system manage to halt this reaction and it is not permanent.

Autoimmunity and MS

Immune cells are active in the MS brain but there does not appear to be an obvious reason for this, such as an infection. This invites the theory that the immune system must be attacking brain tissue because it somehow has mistaken healthy brain cells for a foreign antigen.

The MS lesion shows extensive oligodendrocyte damage and myelin loss along with inflammatory immune activity. Oligodendrocytes are cells that make the myelin that covers other nerve cells. Myelin is an extension of the oligodendrocyte's cell surface that stretches over and wraps around an adjacent nerve. If the oligodendrocyte dies or is damaged, the myelin dies too. Loss of myelin results in malfunction of the associated nerve so that the corresponding function is less effective or even absent. Fortunately, the oligodendrocyte can recover and remyelinate the associated nerve, or a nearby oligodendrocyte may take over the task of myelinating the area, and then a remission occurs.

As mentioned, areas where the myelin is damaged have marked immune system activity. There are T cells, B cells, multiple cytokines, phagocytes, activated microglia, adhesion molecules and other immune players busily working in the area, which eventually becomes scarred.

The favored interpretation of the known facts is that the immune system caused the dead oligodendrocytes and myelin. The following things are widely accepted regarding MS immune system activity and are often referred to as suggestive of an autoimmune process:

1. T cells are present in MS lesions and appear to be targeting myelin. Recall that T cells are activated after being presented with an antigen in a class II MHC. The T cells in the MS lesion are clonally expanded CD8+, meaning they are a result of a focused immune response to a specific antigen.

2. Macrophages are in the area and are full of myelin, meaning they have "eaten" the myelin.

3. The cerebrospinal fluid (CSF) is full of cytokines in the inflammatory TH1 pattern.

4. Activation of immune cells seen in MS lesions is somewhat similar to lesions in experimental autoimmune encephalomyelitis and EAE is a scientifically proven classic autoimmune disease.

5. There is complement in some MS lesions. Recall that complement can be activated several ways. One way is when there is an antibody attached to the cell, marking it for destruction. Complement may also act on its own or in cases of dead or damaged cells.

6. Oligoclonal bands are seen in the CSF of MS patients and these are immunoglobin G, indicating B cell creation of antibodies in the CSF. The antibodies reveal a mature immune response (IgG rather than IgM), which indicates repeat activation against the same antigen.

7. An antigen-driven "highly focused" immune activation is deemed likely because there is evidence of clonally expanded T cell and B cell populations. In one study 30 percent of T cells in an MS lesion had come from a single cell (Hemmer et al. 2002).

Autoimmunity will be considered scientifically proven when the immunological marker (an abnormal immune cell not seen in healthy people that is programmed to attack brain tissue) and antigenic target (the antigen it attacks) are positively identified. But why have they not been able to positively identify this in MS?

Some think that they have. They believe that the T cell is the problem and it is attacking myelin. However, the level of T cells in the lesion is low, and there are far more macrophages; macrophages outnumber T cells by at least 10 to 1 (Barnett et al. 2009a). This suggests that perhaps the immune response is innate because macrophages are key to innate immunity.

An earlier research team makes this comment:

> Many investigations of MBP (myelin basic protein- ed.) reactivity in MS have used 7-day proliferation assays of whole peripheral blood mononuclear cells. These studies have shown a slight increase in T cell responses to human MBP in subjects with MS as compared to normal subjects or other neurologic disease patients, but the magnitude of the difference generally has been less than convincing [Hafler and Windhagen 1995].

It remains a frustrating fact that the T cell autoimmune model remains scientifically unproven (Hemmer et al. 2002). Research comparing the T cell populations in MS patients and healthy people has found that there are no differences that could account for the fact the MS patients have a disease and the others do not.

There is a growing suspicion among researchers that the immune system activity in MS is much more complex than the simple classic autoimmune model (Schwartz and Kipnis 2002). Another speculation is that the problem in MS may be dysregulation of the immune system.

The normal immune system makes myelin-active T cells, as mentioned earlier, but it also makes factors at the same time that are supposed to regulate these T cells (Yoles et al. 2001). In a normal injury to the brain the body makes myelin-active T cells that worsen damage while they begin healing for about a week, and then regulatory cells trigger apoptosis (programmed cell death) in these T cells. Injecting myelin-active T cells into a nerve crush injury results in improved healing; this is part of protective autoimmunity (Kwidzinski et al. 2003).

If the regulatory cells that are supposed to trigger apoptosis are not working properly, then this balance may be upset. Instead of helpful, limited autoimmunity, the result would be damaging autoimmune disease caused by dysregulated controlling factors in the system.

Yet even this sophisticated theory has a problem; few people with MS suffer from additional autoimmune diseases (Somers et al. 2009). Loss of this regulatory mechanism would have to occur only in the CNS for this theory to account for MS autoimmunity alone. It is difficult to understand why this mechanism would function elsewhere in the body but not in the CNS considering the regulatory cells come from the body.

Researchers have generated a lot of data about immune system activation in MS, looking for scientific proof that it is an autoimmune disease. The volume of detailed information leads many physicians to have a sense of certainty about the eventual outcome of this work, though the results remain inconclusive at this point. The uncomfortable scientific fact is that the autoimmune model of MS is unproven.

The MS Process: The Heart of the Issue

One issue hampering understanding of multiple sclerosis is that it is extremely difficult to evaluate what the MS *process* is because it takes place inside the living human brain. The process is the actual sequence of events, not just what the lesion looks like on autopsy. This process needs elucidation.

> Since the earliest lesion in MS is not known, examination of the brains of patients who have had the illness for some time makes it impossible to give a precise age to the inflammatory or demyelinating lesions found. There is still little knowledge as to the precise pathological processes and timing of events that occur in the genesis of the MS plaque [Behan and Chaudhuri 2002].

Discovery of an animal model became critical to early MS research because animals can be sacrificed at all developmental stages of the disease, giving the researcher access to a step-by-step view of lesion development.

Reviewing what is known about EAE and how it relates to MS today is important to understanding how thinking about the cause of MS evolved based on developments in EAE research. It is also important to the big picture of MS research because EAE is not actually MS.

Experimental Autoimmune Encephalomyelitis (EAE)

In chapter 2, EAE was discussed in the context of MS history. The discovery of EAE was a critical event for the development of the autoimmune theory of MS causation.

Initial attempts to develop an animal model of MS in the early twentieth century met with great difficulty. The breakthrough came when researchers understood a rare illness that occurred in a few people after they received a rabies vaccine.

Researchers of the time knew that a rabies vaccine could trigger a temporary illness in some people clinically similar to MS. The desiccated spinal cord tissue used to make the rabies vaccine came from rabbits. This caused some people's immune systems to make myelin antibodies, which attacked the myelin in their brains. This disease, acute disseminated encephalomyelitis (ADEM), is a different disease from MS, although the patients initially have the same symptoms.

ADEM is a temporary neurological illness caused by acute demyelination that does not result in MS plaques or chronic disease. It is a self-limited, one-time event. It is difficult even today for the MD to differentiate the two diseases at initial presentation (Dale and Branson 2005). The rare person who develops ADEM after a virus or vaccination usually recovers without any long-term deficits. It is a classic autoimmune disease (Behan and Chaudhuri 2005).

Early researchers looking for a way to develop animal MS began to think about creating this illness in experimental animals. It was thought that it would be possible to create a true animal multiple sclerosis by starting from a lab-created ADEM.

Mice were altered in many ways in the effort to succeed in creating a type of EAE that would be similar to MS. One way that resulted in a vigorous EAE was genetically altering immune cells so that they would naturally recognize myelin as a foreign tissue and attack it. This was done in one type of mouse by making all the T cells in that animal's immune system carry a genetically inserted receptor for myelin. This meant the immune system was designed to attack myelin naturally. Such mice can develop EAE spontaneously when exposed to bacteria.

Another type of transgenic mouse was designed to express a viral protein (antigen) in its oligodendrocytes. This mouse variety develops EAE when it contracts the virus that matches the viral protein that was inserted into its oligodendrocyte's genetic code; the myelin is attacked just as if it were the virus.

There are many other types of EAE as well. The two mentioned are just examples. These types of EAE were not developed because these anomalies are what is seen in MS patients; instead, researchers were manipulating the mice in an attempt to create an EAE that looks more like human MS.

One might argue that what is thought to be true about MS is actually what is known to be true for EAE. This approach has not resulted in the hoped-for success with multiple sclerosis itself. The few drugs that have come through the EAE pipeline do not stop MS as they do EAE.

> Because specific T-cell mediated autoimmunity can be reproduced in animals after myelin protein sensitization (Experimental Allergic Encephalomyelitis (EAE)) it has been assumed (but never proven) that a similar T-cell driven immune mechanism is responsible for demyelination in MS [Behan and Chaudhuri 2002].

Some researchers have criticized blind reliance on EAE; they have suggested EAE is not as similar to MS as it should be considering the emphasis that is placed on EAE research. Diverse workers from many countries have made that argument in well-referenced and supported peer-reviewed work.

One of these objections is that EAE may arguably be simply an animal model of ADEM (Chaudhuri 2004). EAE, like ADEM, is a self-limiting disorder, meaning the individuals suffering from it recover naturally. Mice typically recover in 7 days. The relapsing or recurring forms of EAE require some type of continual exposure to an antigen or genetic manipulation to develop ongoing disease.

> In contrast to the accepted theory, the human counterpart of the experimental autoimmune demyelinating disease, EAE, is not MS but a different demyelinating disorder, i.e. acute disseminated encephalomyelitis (ADEM) and acute hemorrhagic leukoencephalitis (AHLE). Extrapolation of EAE research to MS has been guided largely by faith and a bland acceptance rather than sound scientific rationale [Behan and Chaudhuri 2002].

The type of immune system activation is different in EAE as well. The cytokines activated are variable in MS, whereas in EAE they are specific to the type of antigen used. The cerebrospinal fluid shows antibodies to myelin in EAE, but rarely is that true in MS (Behan and Chaudhuri 2005). In a paper on macrophage activity which concludes that the activation appears to be scavenging activity and not a primed attack, this statement is made: "Unlike the lesions of EAE, CD4+ T cells are outnumbered by MHC class I restricted clonally expanded CD8+ cells in active MS lesions" (Barnett et al. 2006).

Taken together, these mean that on a cellular level the immune activation is not the same when comparing EAE to MS. Researchers create EAE so they know the cause of the autoimmune inflammatory reaction in the animal model; therefore, these differences at the microscopic level suggest the cause of MS is not the same as EAE.

Another important issue is that white matter in EAE and ADEM are normal; MS white matter is not normal even if it appears to be so. As mentioned in the last chapter, the NAA levels are low in the normal-appearing white matter, showing that nerve damage exists prior to visible changes. There are also fibrin cuffs remote from MS lesions in normal-appearing white matter (Barnett et al. 2006). One research team notes that the progressive brain and spinal cord atrophy, which is significant and the primary cause of disability in MS patients, is not reproduced in EAE (Behan and Chaudhuri 2005).

EAE is easily curable by multiple agents. Sriram and Steiner mention "over 100." For example, glatiramer acetate stops EAE completely. This is not true of MS. More sinisterly, anti–TNF agents (used in rheumatoid arthritis) stop EAE completely but make MS worse. Quoting from the paper, "None of the EAE models represent MS and they therefore are imprecise methods to elucidate either the pathogenesis or to develop therapeutic strategies in MS" (Sriram and Steiner 2005).

In spite of this, EAE is still a useful model for studying inflammation in the brain. The brain has limited ways to respond to damage and inflammation occurs inside the brain in many pathological processes, including MS.

Multiple sclerosis is an inflammatory disease; that is not in dispute. Relapses are proven inflammatory events. The usefulness of EAE is therefore a given when considering some aspects of MS inflammation and damage as long as the limits of that usefulness are respected.

In a paper comparing the virtues and pitfalls of EAE for MS, for instance, the point is made that drugs can be tested in the animal model before trying it on humans (Steinman and Zamvil 2005). This highlights the dilemma that MS researchers find themselves in: they must have a way to test pharmaceuticals before using them on human beings, so they are forced to accept EAE as the best way to avoid human injury even though it is imperfect.

The authors also point out that "despite its pitfalls EAE has been a useful model for predicting clinical success with clinical trials in multiple sclerosis." Both glatiramer acetate and natalizumab were developed using EAE. Both drugs stop EAE and both were later shown to reduce inflammatory lesions and relapses of multiple sclerosis in human trials (Steinman and Zamvil 2005).

Similarities in the two diseases regarding inflammation are thus proven when an approach impacts inflammation in EAE and then the same approach is shown to reduce some indicators of MS damage. One must concede the value of EAE in aiding research aimed at reducing inflammation.

The problem comes when people assume that EAE is the same as MS. Though they share important similarities, the disease process may be completely different.

"The disease process" is at the very heart of the issue. The question is not whether there is inflammation in MS; there is. The real question is this: what starts this process, what is the first event and how does that end in clinical MS? Degeneration and atrophy are prominent and related to progressive disability in human MS and are not well reproduced in EAE. What is the cause of neurodegeneration in human MS?

In spite of the inability to reach scientific certainty about the root cause of MS, therapies are available now that have been shown in clinical trials to reduce inflammatory features of MS. In the next section the autoimmune theories that relate to current standard therapies are briefly discussed.

Selected Autoimmune Theories in MS and Related Pharmaceuticals

Many people in the medical community believe MS is autoimmune. The vast amount of research into EAE and its similarities to MS gives them a feeling that finding proof is just a matter of time. There is clearly extensive inflammatory activity but the trigger for this and exactly how the disease develops have stayed frustratingly out of reach. However, the database generated by people trying to solve the MS puzzle offers some candidates.

What follows are the autoimmune models associated with the most common MS pharmaceuticals, which are prescribed for their ability to suppress inflammatory immune system activity in MS.

General Immune System Suppression

Approaches that suppress immune system activity in general seem to be helpful for some MS symptoms.

The earliest approach that showed success in reducing signs of an MS relapse was to give patients adrenocorticotropic hormone, which caused their adrenal glands to make steroids. Today, steroids themselves, such as methylprednisolone, are given to many patients when they have an exacerbation to reduce symptoms, though it does not help all patients (Visser et al. 2004). Steroids suppress immune function and rapidly reduce inflammation. Recall that inflammatory activity in the lesion is the cause of clinical symptoms when a patient relapses because inflammation causes demyelination and dysfunction of the nerves (Tsutsui and Stys 2009).

By the 1980s it was clear that giving MS patients steroids for a relapse resolved the symptoms much more quickly. Unfortunately, there was no long-term benefit (Nos et al. 2004).

Since steroids impact other bodily functions, patients cannot take them long term. Because of this, researchers developed other approaches to suppress immune function in a broad way that are not steroids.

The drug mitoxantrone is a broad immune system suppressant. It inhibits B cells, T cells, macrophage activity, antigen presentation, tumor necrosis factor-a and interleukin 2 (FDA monograph on Mitoxantrone 2010). This is a very broad suppression of immune activity but it has significant side effects and does not stop MS progression over time, though it may slow it.

Another approach that results in broad immune suppression is alemtuzumab, a drug that is still in trials. This drug was originally created for cancer, but its broad suppression of immune function was thought to make it a candidate for MS. This approach works on the same "reboot the immune system" principle as ASCT but with less toxicity. However, this drug has significant side effects and concerns about safety have kept it in trials, though it seems to have promise with exceptional reduction of inflammatory immune system activity in people still in the inflammatory phase of the disease. It does not help people with progressive disease (Coles et al. 2002).

Autologous stem cell transplant (ASCT) was discussed in chapter 2 within the context of inflammation and degeneration. Recall that it appears that degeneration continues in spite of ASCT eliminating inflammation. This broad suppression of immune activity is based on the concept that a new naïve immune system is not likely to make the same mistake in targeting the brain with autoimmune cells again.

Small studies on ASCT have resulted in scattered findings, but a review of many other studies in 2009 covering about 400 patients who had received ASCT revealed that at 3 years about 70 percent of the patients remained stable (Rogojan and Frederiksen 2009). Another review that evaluated people in a European database revealed that at 3.5 years 63 percent had stabilized or improved (Saccardi et al. 2006).

Another study on ASCT evaluating 26 patients also confirmed that at 3 years 70.2 percent remained stable. However, this group looked at data further out as well; at 6 years the percentage that remained stable had dropped to 29.2 percent (Krasulova et al. 2010). A larger database from a European working group evaluating ASCT in MS listed 45 percent as stable 5 years post-procedure. They also list mortality from treatment for MS patients as 2 percent (Farge et al. 2010).

Across these studies, the patients who did best were under 35 years of age and had MS for less than 5 years, perhaps because they were still in the inflammatory phase of the disease and had not yet reached the age of progression, as discussed in chapter 2. The conclusions of these papers were that ASCT is an important option for patients with very aggressive, malignant MS. ASCT seems to stop inflammatory activity very effectively (Fassas and Mancardi 2008).

All of these approaches that suppress immune function generally appear to be successful at reducing inflammatory activity. Some suppress immune activity to the point where the person must be monitored carefully because a side effect of the drug is vulnerability to infection or cancer (Berger and Houff 2009). A normal immune system is important to health; it cannot be eliminated without consequences. Unfortunately, none of these approaches work well for people already in the progressive phase of MS and none have been proven in randomized controlled trials to stop development of the progressive phase in persons with RRMS. Even scrutinizing ASCT research shows that as time goes on the majority of people do slip into progression. It's the old "inflammation vs. progressive disability" problem rearing its ugly head again.

Myelin-Active T Cells

As mentioned earlier, one of the most commonly accepted hypotheses about the cause of MS is that an unknown factor primes T cells to attack myelin. EAE is caused by myelin-active T cells. In people with MS, there are T cells attacking myelin in the area of active lesions and T cells that react to myelin can sometimes be found in the blood of people with MS (Stinissen and Hellings 2008).

Myelin-reactive T cells (MRTCs) were recently the focus of an experimental approach. The idea was to induce the immune system to eliminate the MRTCs. The working name for this trial drug was Tovaxin (Opexa 2008). The drug was created for each individual person on a case-by-case basis. This was done by taking some blood from the person needing treatment and finding the cells that would react to myelin peptides. Those cells were then altered in a lab to make them "foreign" to the immune system so that the immune system would attack any similar cells. These cells were then given back to the patient in a vaccine.

This elegant approach was designed to eliminate any MRTCs from the person's immune system and *only* those cells, leaving the remaining immune function intact. This would be a huge improvement over broad suppression of the immune system. The assumption was that MS is caused by T cell activity exclusively and this approach would end MS autoimmunity.

Notably, many patients did not have any MRTCs. Such volunteers could not participate in the study.

The IIb clinical trial testing Tovaxin on 150 people with MS was started in 2006, then stopped in 2008. The company announced at that time that it had not reached statistical significance in the primary endpoint, though there was a trend toward positive reductions (Opexa 2008). Later post-hoc analysis revealed more promising findings in endpoints not originally evaluated, such as improvements in EDSS, quality of life scores and annualized relapse rates. Thee researchers are currently seeking funding to continue and refine the approach and have obtained patents for their process. Such an approach, should it be refined, might be expected to minimally impact immunity while still helping to reduce immune system activation in MS.

The weakness in this theory is whether the immune system cell that was chosen by the researchers is actually the one that causes MS autoimmunity.

Another weakness is that trauma in the CNS such as stroke also causes myelin-active T cells to be detectable in the blood. Persons who had a stroke have 7 times the numbers of MRTCs when compared to healthy controls (Barnett et al. 2006). Stroke is not an autoimmune disease, nor does having a stroke result in MS-like autoimmune attacks after the stroke (Kwidzinski et al. 2003). The mere presence of MRTCs is therefore not specific for MS but is found when there is an immune response to damage to the CNS, which calls this theory into question.

Cytokine Dysregulation

The numerous cytokines mentioned earlier have great potential for modulating the immune system. Recall that the T helper cells control the cytokines and regulate immune system activation. It is thought that by nudging the immune system toward a less inflammatory cytokine profile, MS can be ameliorated. Several of the current therapies work in the realm of the cytokines to reduce inflammation.

Adhesion molecules are molecules that make white blood cells stick to the blood vessel and migrate out into the tissue. This makes it possible to repair a wound. For example, if a person had a thorn in the thumb, adhesion molecules would allow immune cells to go from the bloodstream into the thumb tissue. Natalizumab blocks an adhesion molecule. This prevents immune cells from going into the brain in MS. The obvious problem with this is it also blocks helpful immune cell migration, and indeed patients on this drug have a risk of getting PML, an *opportunistic* viral brain infection. Opportunistic means it takes advantage of people with compromised immunity.

Glatiramer acetate was originally thought to be a decoy for the immune attack; it was designed to look like myelin to the immune system. It seems now that it also modulates the immune system by binding strongly with MHC and biasing the profile toward a milder TH2 cytokine profile (Arnon and Aharoni 2004). This results in suppression of inflammation.

The other first-tier approaches to MS are the interferon drugs. Beta interferon is normally produced by fibroblasts and has antiviral effects. Several companies make interferon drugs. Cytokine activity is altered in the following ways by taking an interferon: it reduces antigen presentation and T cell proliferation, alters cytokine expression and restores T suppressor function (Markowitz 2007).

The cytokines are a wide-open field for pharmaceutical intervention to modulate the immune system. There are potentially many other ways in which immune activity can be impacted by altering cytokines and some of these other approaches are currently being investigated in the hope that a more effective drug will be discovered.

All of these approaches have demonstrated signs of reduced inflammatory activity in clinical trials, though no approach to date has been shown to actually stop development of the progressive phase of the disease. But the tantalizing improvements, even though frustratingly small, lead many to feel research is on the right track.

But there is another possibility — that multiple sclerosis may not be a primary autoimmune disease. Evidence compiled by researchers who believe this may be true will be offered in the next section.

Evidence Against the Autoimmune Theory in MS

Franz Schelling, MD, has written a thorough historical account of how the autoimmune hypothesis came to be the leading theory, as well as a critical review of the circumstances that allowed it to become entrenched. His account uses the full scope of the published works from the beginning of MS research in the 1830s to follow the trends and development of MS theory all the way into today.

Dr. Schelling points out that as individual researchers became proponents of individual theories, important facts about the MS lesions that did not fit their ideas were simply ignored. For example, it has been known since the time of Dawson that the lesions exist on veins *of a certain size*, yet this is never accounted for by any theory, as if such a fact does not exist (Schelling 2004, 66). According to Schelling, the systematic ignoring of such facts allowed the propagation of an immunological theory that never did fit the real physical findings. Here is a quote from the book:

> It seems in fact that the present speculative approach to the subject matter, involving the futile quest for some figmentary, in particular immunological, multiple sclerosis agent can be abandoned without scruples. This should be done in all haste to avoid prolonging unnecessary human (and animal) suffering [Schelling 2004, 72].

As discussed earlier, the theory that MS is primarily autoimmune remains unproven from a scientific standpoint. There is a growing body of evidence today that suggests perhaps MS is not initiated by autoimmune activation of the immune system (Barnett and Sutton 2006; Behan and Chaudhuri 2005). Authors from all over the world have contributed to this body of published medical literature.

One of the leading researchers in the field of multiple sclerosis is John Prineas, whose work on the pathology of MS lesions spans 40 years. Much of what is thought to be true about MS has come from his work. In 2009, Dr. Prineas was the recipient of the prestigious Charcot Award for lifetime achievement in multiple sclerosis research. He had previously received the Dystel Prize for MS research.

Dr. Prineas has addressed subjects in his published work as diverse as remyelination of MS lesions in a paper published in 1979 to work in 1985 that suggested MS was primarily degenerative (Prineas 1985), and further work in 1994 that suggested MS appeared to be caused by immunological mechanisms (Prineas 1994). Dr. Prineas is often asked to write chapters for books on the pathology of multiple sclerosis for professionals. He continues today as senior adviser for the NMSS lesion project. This is a researcher whose lifetime achievement has contributed incalculably to our understanding of immune activation in MS.

Yet his recent papers suggest the initiating event in MS may not be an autoimmune attack.

In 2004 Barnett and Prineas published a paper titled "Relapsing and Remitting Multiple Sclerosis: Pathology of the Newly Forming Lesion." In this research they examined the lesions of people who died shortly after an MS relapse. What they discovered was unexpected: it turned out that these early lesions showed extensive oligodendrocyte apoptosis (death) and early signs of microglial activation, but no lymphocytes and no phagocytes attacking the myelin (Barnett and Prineas 2004). This is entirely different from EAE.

The changes seen in the oligodendrocyte were indicative of a special kind of cell death called caspase independent apoptosis (Barnett et al. 2006). Caspase independent apoptosis occurs in nerves when they are damaged by hypoxia, ischemia or excitotoxins (Cregan et al. 2002).

Barnett and Prineas suggest that this phase in which the oligodendrocyte has become apoptotic but the microglia have only just begun to activate is probably only hours long. It is naturally going to be rare for researchers to see the MS lesion in this very brief phase of lesion development.

The discovery of apoptotic oligodendrocytes and no T cells at the scene of the crime is problematic for theories that have their basis in T cell autoimmunity. Recall that the immune system removes dead or damaged tissue. Damage to a cell releases chemo-attractants that bring phagocytes to the area to clean up. The Barnett and Prineas findings suggest the phagocytes were activated in an innate immune response to clean up the apoptotic cell instead of the T cell barging into the CNS and wreaking havoc. The traditional theories have maintained for decades that T cells attack healthy myelin and this is the cause of MS. An apoptotic cell is not healthy. An apoptotic cell is one that naturally attracts immune activity.

The paper does not stand alone; members of the team collaborated with others to replicate the work as well. In 2009 Henderson et al. made this statement:

> Early loss of oligodendrocytes is a prominent feature in tissue bordering rapidly expanding MS lesions. Macrophage activity is largely an innate scavenging response to the presence of degenerate or dead myelin. Adaptive immune activity involving T. and B. cells is conspicuous chiefly in recently demyelinated tissue, which may show signs of oligodendrocyte regeneration. The findings suggest the plaque formation has some basis other than destructive cell-mediated immunity directed against myelin or oligodendrocytes antigen [Henderson et al. 2009].

What this means is that in the opinion of the authors the macrophage activity they observed — in other words, the eating of the tissue by phagocytes — appeared to be innate scavenging and not the result of immune system priming. Such scavenging is, of course, normal when there is dead tissue.

Recall that adaptive immune activity means the specific immune response discussed earlier, which involves activation of T cells and B cells. They felt the adaptive (targeted) immunity activated after the scavenging of the dead tissue, which is a normal sequence of events. The researchers noted these T cells and B cells were present where *regeneration* of oligodendrocytes was occurring. In their view, the T cells and B cells were not the primary drivers of the damage; the areas that showed the presence of the adaptive immune cells were the areas that were healing. Other researchers have noted that T cells are involved in healing as well (Kwidzinski et al. 2003; Yoles et al. 2001).

The borders of rapidly expanding MS lesions show remyelination and healing "shadow plaques," areas with thin, new myelin. These areas are full of macrophages that are full of myelin — in other words, macrophages that ate myelin. Yet they are not eating the new myelin (Prineas 2009). The logical explanation for that is that the old myelin, which they ate, was damaged.

In another study looking at macrophage activity in autopsy samples, another Barnett team of researchers document that *before* the phagocytes/microglia activated the oligodendrocyte became apoptotic and the myelin was altered because of that. They term these alterations pre-phagocytic changes and suggest this may be the very first event in the MS process (Barnett et al. 2006).

The researchers hypothesize that what they saw may be accounted for by transcription of phosphatidylserine in the oligodendrocyte cell surface, which amounts to the "eat me — I need assisted suicide" signal to the phagocytes. The myelin would be greatly affected by this because it is an extension of the oligodendrocyte cell surface — where all the phosphatidylserine is — making myelin a prime target.

It was unclear to these researchers what had caused the death of the oligodendrocyte, though they mentioned the similarity to hypoxia (low oxygen) damage:

> In keeping with this, the pathology that accompanies white matter ischaemia can closely resemble prephagocytic changes in evolving MS lesions and Pattern III pathology. MAG and CNP, proteins concentrated in the distal (adaxonal) myelin membrane, appear to be preferentially lost in such lesions, as is seen in the first days following acute white matter stroke [56], and hypoxia inducible factor (HIF 1 a), a marker of hypoxic tissue injury, is expressed in both lesion types [55]. Lesional oedema, endothelial dysfunction and even immune-mediated microvessel occlusive vasculitis have been proposed as possible contributory factors [Barnett et al. 2006].

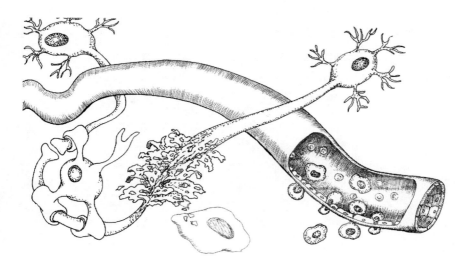

This image is an example of a model of MS causation in which cells die first and inflammation occurs after the fact, such as the one offered by Barnett and Prineas. In their model, they postulate the oligodendrocyte is damaged and undergoes caspase independent apoptosis, causing loss of myelin. This triggers an innate immune response beginning with the microglia. The microglia move to the damaged myelin and initiate the immune response: they eat the dead myelin, then present the antigen of the damaged tissue to the other cells of the immune system. This brings myelin-active T cells and other immune cells across the blood brain barrier (BBB) and into the area to aid cleanup and healing of damaged cells. An important part of such innate immune activity is the macrophages (big eaters). Macrophages outnumber T cells in the MS lesion by at least 10 to 1. Image courtesy of Marv Miller.

What this quote says is that lack of oxygen (ischemia) causes changes that resemble what was seen just before the phagocytes scavenged the damaged oligodendrocyte. They point out that when someone has a stroke, which is a problem with severe low oxygen, the changes in the tissue are similar. This low oxygen state may be caused by fluid in the MS lesion (oedema), failure of the endothelium (walls of the blood vessel) or even tiny blood clots in the micro-vessels. Venous insufficiency and low oxygen levels in the tissue are discussed at length in the next chapter.

Hypoxia is not the only possible cause of oligodendrocyte loss, however. In an interview Dr. Prineas stated he felt the most important development in MS research since EAE was the discovery of a specific autoimmune cell in Devic's disease. This immune cell targets a cell called an astrocyte in the brain and this results in immune activity that causes standby damage to the oligo-dendrocytes and demyelination similar to MS (Prineas 2009). The cause of oligodendrocyte apoptosis as documented in the Barnett et al. 2006 research is not understood yet. It may be an autoimmune loss of some unique sort such as that seen in Devic's, or it may be another factor like hypoxia causing oligodendrocyte loss.

However, the debate over whether MS is a primary autoimmune disease, meaning autoimmunity is the main problem, or if possibly something else initiates the MS process is focused on more than just the possible initiating event. Some people are using deductive reasoning to argue that we are missing something with the autoimmune-centric point of view. Here's a recent comment in *Neurology*:

> Importantly, despite even potent modulation of the immune system, which results in profound reduction of inflammatory lesions, the effect on long-term disability and progression is not as robust as we would expect or hope for, and treatment of progressive disease has thus far been a failure. Curiously, and perhaps counterintuitive to the notion of inflammation as a major driver of progressive disability, relapses do not significantly influence later progression [Tsutsui and Stys 2009].

The "not as robust as we would expect" comment is an important point. Knocking out inflammation should stop eventual progression if autoimmune activation is the cause of progressive MS; the fact that it doesn't suggests the current model is missing something.

If the first event in the MS lesion is oligodendrocyte apoptosis, managing inflammation is not going to change that part of the MS process, although it would reduce inflammatory reaction to that event (Barnett et al. 2009a). Reducing the inflammatory reaction would reduce damage to the brain as inflammation is accompanied by reactive oxygen species, excitotoxicity, and standby damage to nearby nerves. The process-related question is this: If oligodendrocytes are undergoing caspase independent apoptosis, what might be the cause of that? The answer to this question may be the key to MS.

Plain-Language Summary and Comment

The immune system is a complicated cascade of cellular activities. In addition to protecting a person from outside bacteria and viruses, the immune system also heals, removes dead tissue, and maintains the health of every cell of the body. These activities include a low level of controlled autoimmune activity.

MS research has been puzzling over the same immunological questions for decades. Immune cells are undeniably targeting "self" tissue in MS; however, there is nothing significantly different about the MS immune system when compared to healthy people that could account for the disease, and it is natural for the immune system to target self cells in a variety of circumstances. The result is that autoimmunity is scientifically unproven in multiple sclerosis, even though it is widely assumed to be the cause of MS.

Another aspect of multiple sclerosis research that remains frustratingly unclear is that it is not known if MS is primarily an inflammatory disease or primarily degenerative, although both are present from the earliest stage. This is a "chicken or the egg" kind of problem, and in spite of decades of research, the solution to this question remains hidden. There are respected researchers on both sides of this debate.

Although the answer to "which happens first" is unclear, standard multiple sclerosis medications are effective at reducing inflammation, and this is a significant portion of the disease. No matter what the actual first event is, there is a tremendous amount of inflammation in MS.

The hope has always been that suppressing immune function would stop progressive disease in the final analysis. Some researchers theorize that the fact that progressive illness has not stopped with current therapies is due to the fact that better or different suppression of immune cells is needed; it is not generally thought to be damning of the paradigm by proponents of the primary autoimmune theory.

But very aggressive immune system suppression has consequences. Immune system activity is necessary for health and life. Eliminating the immune system has serious implications and results in poor healing, opportunistic infections, and even cancer. Finding a balance between the risks of therapy and the hoped-for benefits has been extremely difficult. To date, no drug has been shown to stop the progressive phase of the disease even though available therapies are very effective at suppressing inflammatory immune cells. This suggests that something is being missed.

Newer research suggests the initiating event in the MS lesion is centered on oligodendrocyte loss without immune cell involvement. This work is unfinished but it suggests that MS may be primarily degenerative with inflammation as a natural secondary event, which begs a new question: what caused the loss of the oligodendrocytes?

CCSVI throws a new angle into MS research. Clearly, the work on immune system function in MS is still pertinent, but some research findings take on a different interpretation when the presence of venous malformations is taken into account.

The next chapter looks at the theory behind CCSVI.

4

CCSVI Theory: MS
as a Vascular Disease

There is only one good, knowledge, and one evil, ignorance — Socrates — posted on TIMS

What if everything traditionally thought to be true about multiple sclerosis is wrong? What if there is nothing wrong with the way the MS immune system functions? What if the immune system is just trying to heal brain cells that became damaged by something else? These are questions on people's minds today based on Dr. Zamboni's vascular research.

The CCSVI theory suggests that venous insufficiency plays a significant role in the MS disease process: specifically, the veins that drain the brain and spinal cord are blocked or damaged and this results in venous insufficiency in the brain. Consequently, the blood does not drain freely, causing reflux and leaving the brain congested, which harms the tissue and reduces oxygen levels, damaging brain cells thus causing the immune system to react. Such a scenario could result in secondary autoimmunity. It's also possible that the immune system activation is simply a natural response to brain tissue trauma.

The research that supports this new idea follows scientific principles and is credible. The person who brought this to the attention of modern medicine is a vascular surgeon and is expert in venous insufficiency. His clarity and flash of insight are changing the world of MS, and patients everywhere are feeling hope, many for the first time in years.

Paolo Zamboni, MD

Paolo Zamboni is a person chosen by history to be the right man, in the right place, with the right background and, critically, the right motivation to see things in a completely new way.

Dr. Zamboni is a professor of medicine at the University of Ferrara in Italy as well as director of their Vascular Diseases Center. The center is a research institution and the mission statement for the group indicates their goal is to advance research in the field of vascular disease so that patients can benefit directly from the best possible care as a result. The members of this coalition are all highly respected, published researchers in the vascular field.

Dr. Zamboni's personal focus of study over 27 years of research has been in the area of venous issues and he has an impressive body of work to his credit. His investigation into the cause of MS he recently published indicates it may well be a venous disease. However, because this is a new concept, readers may wonder what kind of credibility he should be given, since, after all, he is not a neurologist.

When looking at a researcher's peer-reviewed work, it's important to look at their academic credentials, publications and previous contributions to the field. The following review of Dr. Zamboni's curriculum vitae will clarify the arenas in which his expertise is acknowledged.

Dr. Zamboni graduated with a degree in medicine in 1982 at the University of Ferrara. He then was a resident in general surgery from 1982 to 1987. In 1986 he became a fellow in the division of vascular surgery at the University of California at San Francisco. Fellowships are the standard in the United States and Canada for specialty training. Once a person has completed their academic training in a specialty, a fellowship is a chance to work in the field with an experienced physician to gain expertise. By 1992 Dr. Zamboni also received a specialty in vascular surgery from the University of Ferrara in Italy. He has been directly involved in both patient care and research in the vascular field since that time.

Dr. Zamboni wrote a book with French physician Dr. Claude Francesci titled *Principles of Venous Hemodynamics*, published in 2009. He is also the recipient of many honors and awards recognizing his work in the field of venous medicine on a worldwide level. He is truly an international figure in the vascular field of medicine.

Dr. Zamboni's publications prior to his interest in CCSVI included peer-reviewed research on genes and how they influence venous ulcers, mutations of particular genes and how that predicts ulcer healing, what kinds of surgeries help venous ulcers heal, which technique of vein repair is best, how iron impacts the venous ulcer, how the ulcer develops, specific immune cell activation involved in the development of venous ulcers, collateral circulation and many, many more papers on all aspects of venous disease. Dr. Zamboni's background and life work on this subject make him a bona fide expert in the arena of venous insufficiency and chronic venous disease, or CVD.

Dr. Zamboni's grasp of CVD is obviously beyond the level of understanding found in the average physician, or even the average specialist in the field.

The reason this is important is that it is from this extensive background in venous insufficiency and its pathological consequences that Dr. Zamboni speaks when he talks about how venous flow impacts healthy tissue such as he has identified in the case of CCSVI. In the 1860s Charcot recognized and noted enlarged veins adjacent to the MS lesions, but he brushed them aside, thinking they were inconsequential because he simply didn't have the background to understand how those distended veins could be an important clue about the disease. If a person is a specialist in another field and is unfamiliar with the hallmark signs of venous disease, how could they recognize it? Why would anyone expect them to?

When Dr. Zamboni's wife was diagnosed with MS in 1995, he began to look at the body of MS literature in order to understand what was known about this disease that had turned their lives upside down. To his surprise he began to see the signature of venous disease, noting among other things that the lesions of MS are all adjacent to veins and that the lesions expand in the direction opposite the normal blood flow. To Dr. Zamboni, this suggested that there was venous involvement and that a countercurrent, chaotic blood flow was perhaps causing MS damage exactly as seen in his CVD research. He began to contemplate the possibility that a vascular doctor would need to collaborate with a neurologist for the optimal benefit of MS patients.

This man's desire to understand his wife's disease led him to discover what MS specialists missed or ignored for decades: there has always been significant evidence that MS is, at least in part, a venous disease.

Before looking at Dr. Zamboni's MS research, readers will appreciate an opportunity to understand the pertinent points from the venous disease literature because it makes the new MS research much easier to understand. The following section offers the basics on chronic venous disease.

Venous Disease

In order to understand venous disease, it is critical to remember that the vascular system is divided into two halves: arterial and venous. The heart pumps blood into the arteries, which branch off and grow smaller and smaller as they work their way out to the tiny vessels of the capillary bed, where oxygen is exchanged for waste gases. From the capillary bed the veins take the blood back to the heart to be recirculated. Veins get larger as they get closer to the heart. When discussing venous disease, this refers to the half of this system that is veins. Increased pressure in the venous system is unrelated to blood pressure readings taken in the doctor's office, which are related to arteries and tell something about how the heart functions.

After the capillary bed, there is very little residual pulse pressure left. The venous system circulates blood back to the heart mainly by movement: muscle movement, breathing, and valves that keep the blood moving in the right direction toward the heart.

Venous disease occurs when the body's venous drainage is inadequate. The drainage can be inadequate because the veins can't carry enough load — for instance, when the veins are damaged, blocked, twisted or somehow impaired; or it can be when the vein is allowing chaotic blood flow that is refluxing.

A blocked or occluded vein is pretty self-explanatory; the blood can't get through for any of a number of reasons and the result is an increase in venous pressure behind the blockage. Refluxing blood, however, is a new concept to people not familiar with venous insufficiency, and it is critically important to this discussion.

When blood flows in a laminar way down the vein, meaning straight down without any swirls or eddies, the endothelium (the lining of the blood vessel) stays healthy. If there is something like a stenosis partially blocking the blood vessel, or an irregularity, then some of the blood refluxes and the flow becomes a chaotic, churning flow seeking a way out. When this happens, it causes a highly localized increase in venous pressure in the refluxing area, and this damages the function of the endothelium (Zamboni et al. 2008).

When there is either a blocked or a refluxing vein, the vein can't do the job of draining the blood away neatly and efficiently, the endothelium changes, and the area that was supposed to be drained essentially gets sick, and it gets sick in a very predictable and specific way.

The first thing that happens is that the vein itself gets stretched out or varicose. This happens because veins (as opposed to arteries, which are thick and strong because they have muscular walls to contend with the pulse) have very thin, weak walls with little muscle supporting them, so when the blood backs up and they become congested, they readily widen out.

This causes another kind of mischief. Most veins, with the exception of some of the cerebral veins, have valves in them, and these valves are critical to good venous return, so once the vein stretches out, the valve flaps are so far apart that they do not work well, which adds to the problem of venous return. With the valve flaps so far apart, the blood has nothing to hold it back so it slips back down the vein instead of moving toward the heart as it should.

This allows the congestion to build up further inside the vein and because of this there is more pressure in the vein than outside of it. This added pressure causes the stressed endothelium to allow the fluid to migrate out into the tissue. It moves through the vein wall and out into the adjacent extracellular spaces (the space between the cells). If the vein in question is in a leg, the most common site for these kinds of problems, the result is a puffy swollen ankle. If this goes on for some time, then not only will more fluid from the circulation migrate out, but red blood cells will leave as well, followed by immune cells, and that is bad news for the tissue in the area.

Iron in the Tissue and Immune System Activation

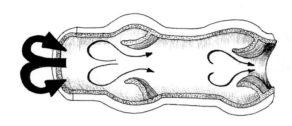

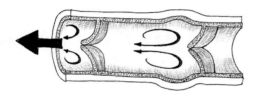

When red blood cells, which have iron in the form of hemoglobin in them, end up in the tissue instead of in the circulation, the immune system cleans it up aggressively because iron can trigger oxidative damage. Iron is important to many different cells and processes inside the body and for this reason the body's iron stores are tightly regulated. Normally, iron is kept in the places where it belongs and removed by the body via the immune system when it is not (Chu et al. 2002; see also Quintana 2007).

This image depicts a healthy vein with laminar blood flow (straight bold arrow) and a distended vein with valves stretched far apart and the swirling chaotic blood flow of reflux. Image courtesy of Marv Miller.

When a person has iron that has been digested by the immune system, it is detectable using current techniques because it changes into hemosiderin. It is the phagocytes that affect this change (Fischbach et al. 1971; see also Chu et al. 2002). Hemosiderin deposits in the tissue are a sign of red-blood-cell leaking of one kind or another — for example, bleeding into the tissue such as in a hemorrhagic stroke — and subsequent phagocyte activity. Even years after a hemorrhagic stroke, MRI can detect hemosiderin deposits in the area where the bleeding previously occurred (Bourgouin et al. 1992).

When the process of converting iron into hemosiderin is going on, hemosiderin can be detected in the urine as the body tries to remove this useless form of iron. People with CVD have hemosiderin in the urine when tested.

Once red blood cells have left the circulation and are in the tissue, the body sends chemical signals to allow the immune system's white blood cells, like macrophages, to sneak out of circulation and into that tissue to do the work of cleaning up the iron. This opening of the endothelium is the task of adhesion molecules.

Adhesion molecules are up-regulated in the case of venous disease, and there are several types of adhesion molecules. They significantly alter the endothelium, the lining of the blood vessels, to allow the white blood cells to migrate out into the tissue. Once the immune system cells are invited into the tissue, a cascade of immune cell activity kicks in that is hard to stop.

This list is taken from a review by Bergan et al. on the changes characteristic of CVD and venous insufficiency:

1. Monocytes and macrophages, which are immune system cells, infiltrate the walls of the vein.
2. ICAMs (intracellular adhesion molecules) and VCAMs (vascular cell adhesion molecules) are up-regulated, which allows white blood cells to migrate.
3. The balance of collagen type changes and there is increased collagen type III compared to type I. Type III makes the vessel more distensible and weaker than type I.
4. Matrix metalloproteinases MMP2 and MMP9 are up-regulated. These break down tissue.
5. TIMP-1, tissue inhibitor of metalloproteinases, is down-regulated, so MMPs are uncontrolled.
6. Integrin is activated, which allows white blood cells to adhere firmly to the vessel wall so migration can occur.
7. T cells and B cells migrate into the tissue to attack and remove damaged tissue.
8. Micro-hemorrhage and tissue death occurs outside the vein.
9. Fibrin pericapillary cuffs form around the vein as an effort at reparative processes.
10. Growth factors TGF-1 (transforming growth factor) and VEGF (vascular endothelilal growth factor) are up-regulated, which thicken some areas of the vein and tissue.
11. The tissue becomes hypoxic from lack of good oxygen exchange.
12. Hemosiderin deposits are prominent in the tissue.
13. The tissue becomes hard and sclerotic — technically, lipodermatosclerosis in CVD (Bergan 2006; see also Alguire and Mathes 2007).

To briefly call attention to how this list of changes in venous disease might relate to MS, recall from last chapter that cytokine dysregulation is one theory for MS autoimmunity. Some dysregulated factors listed above in venous disease (MMP9, TIMP-1, TGF, VEGF, and integrin) are similarly documented as dysregulated in MS. For example, MMP9 has been identified as increased in MS while TIMP-1 is decreased and potentially part of the pathology in multiple sclerosis lesions (Waubant et al. 1999). Similarities between venous disease and MS will be discussed in more depth later in the chapter, but this list of changes in chronic venous disease highlights the inflammatory nature of venous insufficiency.

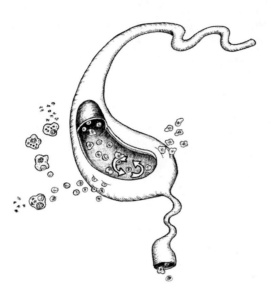

This image depicts a stenosed vein that is experiencing the swirling blood flow of reflux that changes the endothelium. This allows several kinds of cells to leak out into the tissue. Red blood cells, seen here dying in the nearby tissue and degenerating, leave iron behind (black speckles). Macrophages, the big eaters of the immune system, then are responsible for cleaning up the iron and red blood cells misplaced in the tissue. These macrophages become full of iron (speckles inside the macrophages that ate the iron). In addition to this, up-regulation of adhesion molecules like integrin allow other white blood cells to migrate out into the tissue, including T cells, B cells, and monocytes. Cytokine balance is altered, including MMP9 becoming up-regulated and TIMP-1 down-regulating, which allows breakdown of tissue. Transforming growth factor and vascular endothelial growth factor are up-regulated, and these growth factors result in thickened vessel walls termed fibrin cuffs (not shown). In part because of tissue being congested with inflammatory cells and fluid and in part because oxygen-rich blood cannot get into the area via the congested vein, adjacent tissue becomes hypoxic (low in oxygen). Image courtesy of Marv Miller.

Venous specialists recognize the fibrin cuffs and perivenous iron deposits as important signs of venous disease (Brown 2005). While some of the immune activation detailed on the above list can be seen in other inflammatory diseases, the fibrin cuffs and perivenous iron deposits are prominent in CVD and are an important clue to MS possibly being a type of venous insufficiency in the view of Dr. Zamboni (Zamboni 2006).

Venous researchers postulate that iron is particularly toxic to the tissue and causes the tissue to become filled with the by-products of oxidative stress in part because of the immune system activity in the area converting the iron to hemosiderin and attempting to remove it (Allhorn et al. 2003). The oxidative stress is thought to cause even more MMP activation and makes the microenvironment more toxic in a kind of catch-22 that damages more tissue. The immune system activity itself causes a large part of the damage to the tissue in venous disease as it tries to heal the area. Although CVD is not an autoimmune disease, the immune response damages the body and many of the immune cells attack damaged self tissue; in the case of CVD, it is skin tissue that this immune activity targets.

These changes in immune cell activation in CVD are directly traceable back to the changes in blood flow characteristic of venous insufficiency. The pressure in the venous circulation is increased in response to the altered blood flow, which can be either the blockage creating the overall increased pressure in the vein or reflux causing a more localized hypertension and leaking in the area of the refluxing blood flow (Bergan et al. 2006). In both cases the vascular specialist recognizes venous insufficiency because the iron deposits exist in very specific patterns. Unfortunately, the consequences of the vigorous immune activation secondary to this phenomenon are the cause of much of the damage and misery of chronic venous disease as times goes on.

Visible Changes in the Skin

The skin tissue in the ankle is frequently the damaged area when there is venous insufficiency in the femoral vein of the leg. The first visible change is puffiness as the fluid begins to leak out. This may later be accompanied by a brownish discoloration as iron is deposited in the tissue.

However, immune activation at the cellular level is the far more sinister change as the matrix metalloproteinases (MMPs) begin to break the tissue down further and more immune system activity is engendered to clean up iron and dead cells (Raffetto and Khalil 2008). This immune activation, if left unchecked, can result in an actual open lesion, a wound that started from the inside and worked its way out. Chronic venous disease causes lesions that are always surrounded by the brownish discoloration of iron deposits. Iron is a key element to actual lesion formation and tissue degradation (Bergan et al. 2006; Allhorn et al. 2003).

Such wounds can be very difficult and sometimes impossible to heal as the ongoing problem with venous circulation causes continued immune system activity in the area. Another factor complicating healing is that oxygen can't easily get in to the area as a result of the congestion and therefore the area becomes hypoxic (having low oxygen), which further hampers healing (Michiels et al. 2002). Success with these difficult wounds requires diligence and evaluation of all modifiable factors. Restoring circulation is clearly important to restore the hemodynamics so fluid can be removed, immune system activation becomes down-regulated, and oxygen can get in.

Collateral Circulation

When the blood vessel integrity is altered and the ability to carry normal blood volumes is reduced, the body is not completely helpless; it has the ability to initiate collateral circulation (Zamboni et al. 2009a).

Collateral circulation can take several forms, two of which are pertinent to this discussion. First, the body can open up small blood vessels that ordinarily carry tiny amounts of blood so that they expand and can carry a larger volume. This happens when a stenosis blocks a vein and the resulting reflux initiates altered immune cell function locally, which allows the smaller veins in that area to make these changes and expand. The expanded blood vessels then take some of the blood around the blockage, resulting in a partial bypass of the blockage. However, this mechanism of compensation for blocked blood flow is inefficient compared to the original vein (Simka 2009c; Zamboni et al. 2009a).

The other type of collateral circulation is collateral circles, or shunting. Shunting to collateral circles occurs when there is something blocking the normal route for the blood flow and it turns back down the vein to reroute through other existing veins (Francesci 2009). This readily occurs in the body; however, the resulting chaotic, refluxing blood flow alters the normal shear stress in the vein and causes the unhealthy immune cell activation discussed earlier. When diagnostic studies are done and they show a stenosis or other type of blockage accompanied by collateral circulation, this means the restriction to blood flow is significant enough to have initiated the immune cell activation required to cause these changes in what used to be small blood vessels. In both reflux-caused collateral circles and shunting to alternate routes, altered blood flow triggers changes in immune cell activity.

Long Timelines

The changes detailed in this section on venous disease are not necessarily linear. In humans, chronic venous disease can take many years to manifest full-blown venous insufficiency and may never develop to the point of open, non-healing lesions in the skin. There are many factors that may alter the course of venous disease, including genetics, general health, activity level and the ability to be diligent in a conservative treatment regimen including such things as patients putting their feet up for part of the day to enhance venous drainage and compression stockings.

Also, while it is not important to this discussion, interested readers might note that the type of venous insufficiency described here is not the cause of all open lesions of the lower leg; there are other pathologies at work in many and they are beyond the scope of this book.

Main Points: Features of CVD

Chronic venous disease is a serious issue for millions of people. The seemingly minor initial changes hide a dark secret: aggressive immune activity that is damaging the tissue.

Venous insufficiency is well understood in other parts of the body and is characterized by some form of venous hypertension — reflux, a restriction of the vein such as stenosis, or other damage to the vein such as valve damage. Reflux can be just as damaging as gross congestion because of the immune cell activation it causes.

Reflux and chaotic blood flow is followed by iron deposits and gross changes in the activity of adhesion molecules and endothelium, which in turn results in immune cell activation and oxidative damage in the tissue adjacent to the congested veins. Iron deposits surround venous ulcers and the associated damaged vein. The end result is aggressive immune cell activity that changes and permanently damages the tissue affected by it, which, in the case of skin, causes hardened sclerotic dermal tissue and even open lesions that may not heal. These processes take many years and are not linear.

Congestion, collateral circulation and reflux that cause these changes are detectable using today's advanced diagnostics. Iron deposits are also detectable; it is possible to diagnose venous insufficiency by looking at blood flow and the pattern of iron deposition.

It is also clear that the first of defense is removing the cause of this sequence of events to the extent that it is technically possible. Restoring laminar blood flow will allow the best chance at healing because it will allow down-regulation of the immune system activity and return to homeostasis. Doing such an intervention early before these changes are permanent is critical to a good outcome.

However, leaders in the vascular field believe that controlling the inflammation and immune cell activation brought on by the iron misplaced in the tissue is the next frontier for therapeutic approaches in venous insufficiency as much of the damage is caused by immune system activation. The future care of patients with venous disease is projected to be a combination of surgery and immune system management (Bergan et al. 2006; see also Zhang et al. 2007b; Rafetto and Khalil 2008). To a large extent, the damage in CVD is damage to the body caused by the immune system activation, not directly caused by mechanical forces.

When considering the similarities between chronic venous disease and multiple sclerosis, one wonders about the possibility that venous insufficiency and the immune activation that it causes could possibly be mistaken for autoimmune activity at the cellular level. Another question this information raises is whether venous insufficiency and the immune activation it causes might trigger a self-perpetuating autoimmunity.

The next section discusses in depth the initial clues Dr. Zamboni noticed that caused him to form the opinion that MS may actually be associated with venous insufficiency of the cerebrospinal system.

Dr. Zamboni and the Big Idea

In July 2006, nine years after his wife's diagnosis with MS, Dr. Zamboni gave a lecture at the Royal Society of Medicine presenting the theory that MS may actually be a venous disease based on his study of the subject. This lecture was later published in their journal (Zamboni 2006). The hypothesis presented in this paper forms the backbone for the whole venous model.

In this paper, titled "The Big Idea: Iron-Dependent Inflammation in Venous Disease and Proposed Parallels in Multiple Sclerosis," Dr. Zamboni describes the evidence that caused him to suspect that multiple sclerosis could be a form of chronic venous disease resulting from a type of venous insufficiency that he labeled CCSVI. In this section this paper will be quoted extensively. The reader is encouraged to obtain a copy free online and read Dr. Zamboni's words directly (http://foundazionehilarescere.org).

The paper is well referenced and makes the case that MS and CVD are perhaps the same disease process carried out on different tissue: skin in CVD and brain cells in MS. One of the most critical clues for Dr. Zamboni that MS might be a type of venous insufficiency was that perivenous cuffs are present in both MS and CVD. Current medical literature in each field suggests that they are attempts at reparative processes. While many inflammatory diseases have similar types of immune activation, Dr. Zamboni notes that perivenous cuffs are a specific finding that indicates to the venous specialist that there is a venous origin.

MS lesions are found almost exclusively around the small veins, or venules. The lesions themselves expand in the direction opposite normal physiologic blood flow. Dr. Zamboni suggests the hemodynamics of the cerebrospinal system should be investigated, as it may mean that the normal direction of blood flow is altered. This important clue is key to seeing MS as a type of venous insufficiency since lesion development countercurrent to normal physiologic blood flow is a hallmark of venous insufficiency.

Another important clue that can be seen in the MS literature is that the blood-brain barrier, which is a type of endothelium with special tight junctions, always breaks down and leaks just before a lesion begins. Fluid leaking into the tissue prior to lesion formation also marks chronic venous disease.

Dr. Zamboni notes that it is well documented that there is inflammation around the veins in both MS and CVD. He also notes that red blood cells extravasate, or leak out, in CVD and there is evidence this happens in MS as well. There are hemosiderin deposits in both diseases in the affected tissue. Hemosiderin is a by-product of the immune system breaking down iron after it has leaked into tissue (Fischbach et al. 1971).

He also notes similarities in the immune system activity. Adhesion molecules are up-regulated and the white blood cells, a part of the immune system, are activated in both diseases. MMPs (matrix metalloproteinases) are hyperactivated and TIMP-1 (tissue inhibitor of metalloproteinases) is hypo-activated in both diseases, resulting in an imbalance and MMP damage to tissue. MMPs break down proteins and result in tissue destruction.

Another aspect of immune system activity in these diseases is that macrophages and T cells migrate out of the circulation and into the tissue, and macrophages in both diseases are filled with iron. There is a local iron overload in both diseases as well. Dr. Zamboni also notes that there is some suggestion that an HFE mutation, which is a gene associated with how the body handles iron, is altered in both diseases. While iron deposits are seen in other inflammatory disease states, in CVD and in MS the iron deposits are anatomically associated with the veins specifically.

The following table discusses known features of MS and CVD. This table is adapted from one in Dr. Zamboni's paper (used with permission) though his version included numerous references.

Common Findings of the Inflammatory Chain in CVD and MS

Finding	*CVD*	*Multiple sclerosis*
Altered venous hemodynamics	+	?
Perivenous inflammation	+	+
Erythrocyte extravasation	+	+
Hemosiderin deposits	+	+
Adhesion molecule and white cell activation	+	+
Macrophage migration-infiltration	+	+
T cell migration-infiltration	+	+

Finding	*CVD*	*Multiple sclerosis*
Iron laden–macrophage	+	+
MMP hyper-activation	+	+
TIMP hypo-expression	+	+
Local iron overload	+	+
Urine hemosiderin test	+	+
HFE mutation	+	+
Fibrin cuff (ongoing reparative process)	+	+

This group of facts as presented by Dr. Zamboni in his published paper suggests it is possible that MS and chronic venous disease share a similar disease process. Critically important is that these facts demand investigation into the hemodynamics of the cerebrospinal system since it is known that in CVD these changes are caused by venous insufficiency and that by removing venous insufficiency the immune activation and damage to tissue is reduced.

To sum up this key paper, Dr. Zamboni uses research from the field of MS to demonstrate that the clues to MS being a venous disease exist in the published literature. It also drives home the point that the hemodynamics of the cerebrospinal system had not been investigated previous to this work and that there was a critical need for such investigation to check for a venous problem in MS patients.

The existing body of MS literature is extensive and holds a tremendous amount of information regarding immune activation and MS lesion formation. The next section looks at some of this literature that supports Dr. Zamboni's big idea.

MS Literature Seen from the Perspective of CCSVI

As was mentioned in chapter 2, Charcot is considered the father of neurology because his research into neurological disease, including actual autopsy findings, established the first scientific knowledge base about the brain and diseases thereof. He even noted in his circa 1880s illustration of MS plaques the venocentric nature of these lesions as well as the widened perivascular (literally, around the veins) spaces (Schelling 2004, 8).

Unfortunately, Charcot's point of view was that the arterial half of the vascular system mattered, but the venous half was unimportant. Neurology was just finding itself as a field, but even in the nineteenth century, stroke was described well enough for doctors to understand the critical role of the arteries in the delivery of oxygen to cells. Therefore from the earliest day there was a commitment to understanding and improving arterial circulation to make sure of the delivery the oxygen-rich blood to the brain, but there was no interest in the role venous return played in circulatory health. It was incorrectly assumed that once the oxygen had been delivered the return of venous blood was simply immaterial; venous blood would make its way back to the heart somehow and how it did that was not important. The fact that MS lesions were all located on widened veins was duly noted, then put aside as an inconsequential finding of no real relevance.

As was discussed in the section on MS history, other early researchers also noted the venous association of MS lesions. Lack of effective diagnostics in earlier times eventually resulted in researchers dropping that line of inquiry as the field of immunology took center stage. It is clear the idea of MS as a vascular disease is not new, although new technology has offered new tools and diagnostics for evaluating it in a brand new way today.

Modern Science and Evidence of Vascular Pathology

In the mid–1960s a Danish researcher, Torben Fog, did in-depth autopsy work on MS patients showing the fact that the lesions were on veins and that the lesions expanded along the vein, growing opposite the direction of blood flow (Fog 1965). He thus established in modern science, using current techniques and equipment, that MS is a venocentric disease.

This is important because if MS were purely autoimmune, it is hard to understand how the activated T cells and macrophages would select only veins of a certain size for their activity. EAE shows a different pattern of damage, and the borders of the lesion are poorly defined, whereas in multiple sclerosis the borders are highly demarcated (Behan and Chaudhuri 2005). In a paper looking at 95 lesions via MRV (magnetic resonance venography), which shows veins specifically, all but one lesion was on a vein (Tan et al. 2000). There is no certain explanation for MS being so strictly venocentric and localized in the autoimmune model; therefore any new information that suggests a physiologic reason for this must be taken very seriously.

More recent work has also supported the idea that perhaps MS has a vascular component. A good example is that the mean transit time of the blood in the MS brain is very slow compared to normal people. A paper from 2004 by Law and colleagues found that patients with MS had blood flow that was roughly half the speed and they moved roughly half as much blood through the brain when compared to normal people (Law et al. 2004).

It is interesting to note that while the blood flow was slow in MS, the blood *volume* was the same, so the blood was getting in, but somehow it wasn't moving through and out normally. The researchers had no conclusive answer for why this was so.

In another example of research into blood flow looking at differences between PPMS and RRMS using a 3T MRI and dynamic susceptibility contrast, not only did the RRMS patients have significantly slower blood flow than normal people, but in PPMS it was even slower (Adhya et al. 2006).

These researchers were checking flow in the normal-appearing white matter rather than the MS-scarred area, which means the blood vessels they were looking at were not surrounded by hardened, sclerotic MS lesion tissue. MS lesions are physically hard and un-giving tissue, so blood vessels in areas of MS lesions may be unable to expand normally, which might skew the results. The fact that slowed circulation was happening in normal-appearing white matter makes it an especially important finding.

Normal-appearing is a misleading term when discussing MS because researchers have determined the normal-appearing white matter is actually abnormal. This tissue is leaky.

Leaky Vessels

In normal-appearing white matter, the diffusion of water molecules out of the blood vessel and through the blood-brain barrier is increased before the lesion develops. Researchers tested this by looking with MRI at normal-appearing white matter on both sides of the brain, then looking back at what had changed on the side that developed a lesion. It turned out that the side that allowed water molecules to diffuse across the endothelium, essentially a leaky area, was the location of a new enhancing MS lesion. The techniques used by this research team detected changes in their identified diffusion parameters even before the blood-brain barrier breakdown. So, normal-appearing white matter that has veins that allow serum to leak out is the area where a lesion develops (Wuerful et al. 2004).

It has long been a matter of scientific debate and curiosity as to why the blood-brain barrier (BBB) allows diffusion of fluid into the brain tissue in MS. Some suggest perhaps the whole problem in multiple sclerosis is failure of the BBB to remain closed, assuming that the opening of the BBB is the event that allows autoimmunity to occur because formerly sequestered brain tissue is suddenly exposed to the peripheral immune system. Based on this theory, it has been postulated that if only the BBB would remain closed, MS might never happen.

It may be that up-regulation of ICAM-1 (intercellular adhesion molecule 1), which is known to occur in venous insufficiency, is also the reason for the BBB to have opened, since the BBB is simply endothelial tissue with tight junctions. One researcher hypothesizes that perhaps venous insufficiency and reflux in the cerebrospinal system triggers autoimmunity by opening the sequestered brain tissue to the peripheral immune system via the ICAM-1 mechanism (Simka 2009c).

In MS, it is leaking veins specifically that end up with enhancing lesions, and previous MS research has indicated that the tissue of the brain shows a picture of immune cell activity with monocytes and macrophages crossing the BBB (Hemmer et al. 2002). This seems to resemble that of venous disease when compared to CVD research findings discussed earlier. In CVD, the crossing of the endothelium by these immune cells is widely understood to be a result of venous insufficiency, while in MS the mechanism remains speculative.

These facts in the MS literature do not clearly favor the traditional autoimmune theory over this new model that suggests venous insufficiency is a critical factor to understand and consider. It is also possible these two factors interact in a negative synergy to create MS.

Iron: The Key

The question of iron in the tissue of MS brains is one of critical relevance to this new model. While iron might be noted in other neurological diseases — for example, Alzheimer's — it is not specifically perivenous.

A prominent MS researcher, Steven LeVine, evaluated iron in MS and Alzheimer's brains because iron promotes oxidative damage. The hypothesis was that perhaps iron plays a role in the pathology. LeVine notes that in Alzheimer's the iron is essentially in the amyloid deposit (amyloid is the type of lesion in Alzheimer's); in MS he documents that it is found in macrophages, reactive microglia and ameboid microglia, all of which are immune cells. He also mentions macrophages full of iron deposits specifically around the blood vessel in MS: "Round macrophages typically with high concentrations of iron, were present in 4/5 MS brains; they were found adjacent to labeled microglia in white matter devoid of other labeled microglia and/or adjacent to vessels" (LeVine 1997).

The macrophage, an immune system cell, appears to be cleaning up the iron in MS, which is what it does in CVD. In Alzheimer's, iron was detected in neurons and cortices and was thought to be from mitochondria or amyloid deposits. The pattern of iron deposits in these two diseases is not the same and this suggests the iron's presence in Alzheimer's was a result of damage to the nerves themselves by the disease process, while the pattern seen in MS supports Dr. Zamboni's hypothesis.

Another researcher notes that iron and hemosiderin in MS brains are specifically related to veins. He documents signs of hemorrhage both old and new in areas next to the veins as well as fibrin deposits "The multiple sclerosis cases showed venous intramural fibrinoid deposition (7%), recent hemorrhages (17%), old hemorrhages revealed by haemosiderin deposition (30%), thrombosis (6%) and thickened veins (19%). In all, 41% of all multiple sclerosis cases showed some evidence of vein damage" (Adams 1988).

He comments that this iron deposition is different than expected, with more excessive damage to the veins than anticipated from a chronic inflammatory disease. His conclusion is that this constitutes a form of vasculitis, which is to say chronic inflammation and damage of the vein wall itself.

Additionally, some researchers note that the MS lesion specifically appears to be surrounded by iron deposits in the form of hemosiderin. One research team suggests that a possible source of this iron deposition is extravasated blood (Craelius et al. 1982). A similar pattern is seen in CVD: all venous lesions have a brownish ring of iron deposits in the skin surrounding them and extravasated (leaked out) blood is the source of these iron deposits (Bergan et al. 2006). The earliest researchers looking at MS lesions in the 1830s, Carswell and Cruveilhier, noted the peculiar lesion color, documenting that MS lesions appeared to be "brownish" and "reddish grey spots" respectively (Schelling 2004, 6).

Iron that is in the ferrous form is "a chemically irrefutable source of oxidative stress because it is able to catalyze the formation of free radicals via the Fenton reaction" (Quintana 2007). Oxidative damage caused by free radicals is a significant part of MS lesion pathology and degenerative changes (Vladmirova et al. 1998).

It is worth noting that other processes known to occur in the MS brain also contribute to the iron load. The death of neural tissue will result in the release of additional loads of iron; many neurodegenerative diseases show iron deposits in the brain, such as Alzheimer's (as mentioned earlier).

Oligodendrocytes themselves contain a very large amount of iron naturally (Quintana 2007). Oligodendrocytes die in multiple sclerosis and macrophages are in the brain cleaning up the dead tissue. This includes iron. When macrophages are attracted into the area they ingest the free iron and become loaded with iron themselves, thus increasing local iron content further. This can become a self-sustaining inflammatory process because iron is very irritating to the tissue (Haacke 2010b).

In a paper on how iron impacts T cell regulation and apoptosis in both MS and CVD, one researcher speculates that iron perhaps modulates and exaggerates the immune process because it may allow T cells to live on beyond their normal lifespan (Simka 2008). This suggests a possible way for the iron to facilitate autoimmunity because when T cells are done with their reparative work they should naturally die (Kwidzinski 2003).

Newer work on iron and disability in *Neurology* concludes that alterations in iron metabolism can be detected with sonography, then used to predict progression in MS. Higher stores of iron correlate to a poorer outcome: "Conclusions: Neurodegenerative disease — like deep gray matter lesions can be frequently detected by transcranial sonography (TCS) in patients with multiple sclerosis (MS). Findings suggest that TCS shows changes of brain iron metabolism which correlate with future progress of MS" (Walter et al. 2009).

Many researchers have shown that iron deposits in the brain correlate with disability (Zhang et al. 2007a; Bakshi et al. 2002; Neema et al. 2009; Hammond et al. 2008). Current clinical trials focus on lesion load rather than iron deposits, though some researchers have suggested that iron deposits could be considered a surrogate marker for MS (Bakshi et al. 2002; Neema et al. 2009; see also Zhang et al. 2007a).

The term "surrogate marker" means something that can be measured and seen on a diagnostic and is thought to have predictive value for the disease. Lesion loads have been widely accepted as a surrogate marker for MS because they are easily seen on MRI and can be regularly imaged.

Iron deposits are more difficult to evaluate and the current autoimmune model considers the presence of iron to be a simple side effect of the death of nerve tissue rather than related to the pathological process. Researchers arguing against the venous model have insisted that their interpretation of the presence of iron is correct and this disproves the CCSVI theory (AAN 2010, 17). However, if venous disease were part of the MS process, there would be iron deposits from both sources: some deposits similar to what is seen in chronic venous disease and other deposits due to the death of nerve tissue.

Since iron is a key instigator of much of the damage in chronic venous disease in the legs, the acknowledged presence of iron in the area of the brain with MS pathology lends support to Zamboni's big idea and should suggest that interested people keep an open mind about the possibility that iron is part of a pathological venous process rather than exclusively an *epiphenomenon* (a side issue not related to cause) caused by nerve death. A comment in a recent paper suggests this is the right attitude to adopt.

> Future longitudinal studies in a larger population of patients should evaluate iron as a predictor of basal ganglia atrophy, EDSS progression, and neuropsychological test performance to establish whether iron is primary to and causes MS pathology, or whether iron is secondary to MS pathology and simply results from years or decades of inflammatory and neurodegenerative insults [Hammond et al. 2008].

Iron is an important clue that perhaps MS and CVD processes are similar. Supporting this idea, a recent paper specifically looking at iron in the brains of people with MS stated, "Conclusion: Iron may serve as a biomarker of venous vascular damage in multiple sclerosis. The backward iron accumulation pattern seen in the basal ganglia, thalamus and midbrain of most MS patients is consistent with the hypothesis of venous hypertension" (Haacke 2010d).

E. Mark Haacke, PhD, a leading researcher in the field of MRI with a special focus on iron in the brain, feels that there is good evidence that his observations show this backward accumulation of iron along the veins in the basal ganglia and pulvinar thalamus (structures in the deep gray matter of the brain) of MS patients. This iron accumulation may be related to reflux. However, he cautions that the scientific evidence for iron deposits being related to venous reflux, as opposed to buildup of iron from other sources, is not yet confirmed in cadaver brain studies. Further, the iron he sees in MS lesions could be in the form of either hemosiderin from local vascular breakdown or ferritin in the oligodendrocytes from myelin breakdown. In both cases iron is present.

Another group of researchers looking at the issue of iron in the brain of MS patients made this concluding remark: "The findings from this pilot study suggest that CCSVI may be an important mechanism related to iron deposition in the brain parenchyma of MS patients. In turn, iron deposition, as measured by SWI, is a modest-to-strong predictor of disability and progression, lesion volume accumulation and atrophy development in patients with MS" (Zivainidov et al. 2010)

The CNS Is Special

CVD and MS have similarities with regards to iron deposits and the presence of fibrin cuffs; also, the kind of immune system activation seen is suggestive of a similar pathology. However, the cells of the central nervous system (CNS) are very different from cells in dermal tissue. This means there would necessarily be differences in microscopic presentation and type of immune activity.

The CNS is thought to be protected from the peripheral immune system by the blood-brain barrier. This is nothing more than endothelium with special tight junctions to prevent things in circulation from contact with the delicate CNS tissue.

However, the BBB is not impenetrable by the peripheral immune system; in stroke and trauma to the spinal cord the body makes myelin-reactive T cells. During these types of trauma to the CNS, the BBB is open and the peripheral immune cells are allowed in so the dead and damaged myelin can be scavenged and removed.

This occurs readily when there is damage to the cells of the CNS because the resident immune cells of the CNS, a type of macrophage called microglia, have the ability to activate and call the peripheral immune system into the brain using chemical messengers like adhesion molecules. If iron has leaked into the CNS through micro-hemorrhage, then microglia would activate to facilitate the conversion of the iron into hemosiderin just as it does after a stroke. In no way does the BBB prevent peripheral immune system activation in the case of damage to CNS tissue. This is important because it means that if there is damage to the CNS tissue, then peripheral immune activation is expected, even including myelin-reactive T cells. Recall that after a stroke myelin-reactive T cell populations increase seven-fold (Barnett et al. 2006).

But note that the specialized immune cells in the CNS, microglia, do not exist in dermal tissue. Therefore up-regulation and activation of microglia can only be seen in CNS damage and would never be noted in CVD. This means that venous insufficiency in the CNS will be different immunologically and there will be different findings; they will not be identical, even if the triggering pathology is the same. Microglia and the BBB are unique.

Other types of specialized cells exist in the CNS as well. One pair of these is oligodendrocytes and myelin, and these are very prominent in MS literature because the myelin is made by oligodendrocytes and both are damaged very specifically in MS. Myelin is critical to the function of the nerve cells they surround, so loss of myelin results in loss of function. This is at the heart of MS disability.

Hypoxia and Oligodendrocytes

In addition to the solid evidence that iron is a key part of the pathology in MS damage, another area of interest is that the MS brain shows signs of hypoxia, which means low oxygen levels. A study on MS brains details how susceptibility weighted imaging was used to assess cerebral venous oxygen levels and it showed that, compared to normal subjects, MS patients exhibited low oxygen levels (Ge et al. 2009). Blood circulating at half the speed of that in normal persons is one mechanism that may be to blame for this problem in MS (Law et al. 2004). Another possibility is that refluxing blood lowers oxygen levels by reverting lower oxygen blood countercurrent back up the vein. The blood flow, and its impact on oxygenation, needs to be evaluated and considered in research taking into account the possibility of CCSVI.

Another researcher, Lassmann, detailed the similarities between the hypoxia-like damage of MS lesions and white matter stroke, which is an arterial problem. He mentions that some type of vascular pathology could be the cause of this finding in MS. Here is a quote from his paper:

> In this review, evidence is discussed, which show that in a subset of multiple sclerosis patients the central nervous system (CNS) lesions show profound similarities to tissue alterations found in acute white matter stroke, thus sug-

gesting that a hypoxia-like metabolic injury is a pathogenetic component in a subset of inflammatory brain lesions. Both vascular pathology as well as metabolic disturbances induced by toxins of activated macrophages and microglia may be responsible for such lesions in multiple sclerosis [Lassmann 2003].

There is also evidence of hypoxic damage in MS lesions; a marker for hypoxic damage called hypoxia-induced factor is present in MS lesions (Barnett et al. 2006). This can also be seen in stroke lesions, the classic hypoxic brain injury. Recall that in CVD, hypoxia is part of the disease picture and in that case it is known to be because of the altered hemodynamics and venous congestion (Michiels et al. 2002).

There is a connection between low oxygen levels and oligodendrocyte damage; it is known that transient ischemia, which is a situation where there are very low oxygen levels for a short period of time, can cause selective oligodendrocyte death and then loss of myelin while other glial cells survive. In one study, researchers were subjecting lab animals to 10 minutes of 10 percent oxygen (air is 21 percent) to elicit this oligodendrocyte damage for their research (Petito et al. 1998).

Clearly there is evidence that there are low oxygen levels in MS and also that low oxygen levels selectively damage oligodendrocytes and myelin. As was mentioned in the previous chapter, hypoxic damage is one proposed mechanism for the cause of death in oligodendrocytes that was observed in MS lesions by a prominent MS research team. They documented caspase independent oligodendrocyte death before immune cells arrived, calling these *pre-phagocytic* (before the immune system's phagocytes activate) changes (Barnett et al. 2006). Caspase independent apoptosis can be caused by ischemia, hypoxia or excitotoxins (Cregan et al. 2002). The presence of low oxygen states in the MS brain may mean this hypoxia causes the loss of myelin and oligodendrocytes. Since hypoxia is prominent in venous disease, this is another clue that Dr. Zamboni could be on the right track.

In addition to low oxygen levels, other factors damage oligodendrocytes as well. Many books on MS give the impression that oligodendrocyte death and myelin loss is unique to MS. In fact, this is incorrect. Here is a quote from McTigue and Tripathi in their review on oligodendrocytes and factors that impact them:

> [Oligodendrocytes] and their precursors are very vulnerable to conditions common to CNS injury and disease sites, such as inflammation, oxidative stress, and elevated glutamate levels leading to excitotoxicity. Thus, these cells become dysfunctional or die in multiple pathologies, including Alzheimer's disease, spinal cord injury, Parkinson's disease, ischemia, and hypoxia [McTigue and Tripathi 2008].

Pathologists even in the very early days of MS research noted that myelin and oligodendrocyte loss is not exclusive to multiple sclerosis. Multiple findings beginning in the late 1800s showed that demyelination is common in any kind of trauma that results in edema (fluid in the tissue) in the central nervous system (Schelling 2004, 31).

Venous insufficiency results in hypoxia, inflammation and oxidative stress in skin tissue; if there was venous insufficiency in the MS cerebrospinal system, these three factors would be present and potentially harming oligodendrocytes. Elevated glutamate levels, present in MS (Srinivasan el al. 2005), are specifically harmful to nerves because it damages them by a unique pathology called excitotoxicity. Excitotoxicity is common in many types of CNS injury, as the previous McTigue and Tripathi quote alluded.

Additionally, iron itself is known to trigger oxidative stress in oligodendrocytes, which causes damage, demyelination and loss of function: "The oligodendrocyte response to oxidative stress derived from the excess of free ferrous iron would be the lipid damage and demyelination with the consequent perturbation of information transfer [Quintana 2007].

There are clearly multiple ways for the oligodendrocytes and myelin to be lost if MS is a version of venous insufficiency, assuming such venous insufficiency would cause changes in the MS brain that are similar to those known to occur in CVD.

Plain-Language Summary and Comment

The question posed in the early part of this chapter was whether the hypothesis presented by Dr. Zamboni's big idea was justified. The materials selected for this chapter support this hypothesis that venous insufficiency possibly plays a significant role in multiple sclerosis pathology.

There are interesting parallels between venous insufficiency and known facts about multiple sclerosis. Immune system activity is well documented and understood in chronic venous disease and is very similar to that which is seen in multiple sclerosis lesions. Additionally, recent research in venous disease of the lower limbs suggests that suppressing immune system activity may aid healing because immune system activity causes most of the damage, not mechanical forces. If MS is a type of venous disease, it's not at all surprising that immune system activity has been the focus of research; immune system activity is a big problem in both diseases.

From a historical standpoint, the venous changes in multiple sclerosis were considered to be a result of the disease and not significant. Instead, the fact that MS lesions are seen on veins was explained as merely reflecting the fact that immune system cells came from the circulation. Researchers neglected clues that MS might have a significant venous component as if unimportant, such as the fact that all MS lesions are on venules of a very specific size and the lesions grow countercurrent to the blood flow.

Modern-day literature also holds clues that MS could be a venous disease. The mean transit time of the blood in circulation in the brain in MS patients is very slow when compared to that of normal people — less than half the speed in one study. This is very easy to explain in relation to venous insufficiency and difficult if one assumes the cause of MS is exclusively an autoimmune attack. Another clue that MS is potentially a venous disease is that fluid leaks out of the vein that will later develop a lesion. The lesions of venous insufficiency also begin with fluid crossing the endothelium.

With regards to iron, multiple studies have shown that iron loads in the MS brain are associated with progressive disease and higher EDSS scores. Degeneration of nerve tissue results in iron deposits in many neurological diseases because nerve tissue contains a lot of iron, and when nerves degenerate they leave iron behind. Although many neurological diseases result in iron deposits, what's special about multiple sclerosis is that there is iron specifically around the veins and macrophages found in the MS brain are full of iron. This means that these immune cells ate the iron in an attempt to clean up. This pattern is not seen in other neurological diseases, such as Alzheimer's, but is seen in venous disease.

Another factor that lends weight to the idea that at least part of the MS process is related to venous issues is that hemosiderin deposits are present in patients with MS; the presence of hemosiderin is related to red blood cells extravasating out of circulation and consequent immune system activity to degrade the misplaced iron. Iron that degrades without the aid of immune system activity is sequestered in the form of ferritin. Both forms are visible on MRI without any way to discern one from the other, which means that "iron" in the brain as seen on MRI may be either. If MS has a venous component, it is likely both types are present.

Recent work shows that iron is deposited countercurrent to blood flow in the deep structures of the brain. This seems to affirm the observation by Fog that lesions expand in successive waves countercurrent to the blood flow. This countercurrent lesion activity was a key tipoff for Dr. Zamboni that MS could be triggered by venous pathology. Lesions in EAE, a proven autoimmune disease, do not expand in this way at all.

The oligodendrocytes and myelin are very vulnerable to factors that are known to be present in venous insufficiency. Low oxygen, edema, and immune system activity as well as presence of free iron, all of which are present in venous insufficiency, may potentially be the cause of oligodendrocyte loss and demyelination seen in MS.

Opening of the blood-brain barrier has long been an area of scientific curiosity in MS research because the healthy brain should have a closed blood-brain barrier, which keeps peripheral immune system cells out. Venous disease alters the endothelium and allows immune system cells to migrate into the tissue. If MS were a type of venous insufficiency, this could explain why immune system cells are allowed into the brain when they should not be.

Very recent work by Barnett and Prineas looking at newly formed MS lesions (mentioned in the previous chapter) found that oligodendrocytes were dead before the immune system cells had arrived. They later published a paper specifically mentioning hypoxic damage and caspase independent apoptosis as the possible culprit. Since venous insufficiency is known to cause hypoxia, this could possibly play a role in the form of apoptosis that the researchers noted.

It is easy to see that Dr. Zamboni's work may provide insight into some peculiarities that have been unanswered by the model of MS causation that holds multiple sclerosis is purely an autoimmune disease. It is important to recognize the existing MS literature does support a possible role for CCSVI in the MS process and more research is warranted. While most of the literature cited in this chapter supports an association between a venous component and multiple sclerosis, much more research will need to be done before it's clear whether the venous component is just a complicating co-factor that makes MS worse or if it might be causative.

Researchers must take steps to aggressively investigate the venous component of multiple sclerosis. The intriguing clues in the multiple sclerosis evidence base regarding the venous aspects of MS must be built upon to uncover the full scope of the venous aspect of the disease. The whole problem of MS must be reevaluated with a fresh eye, taking into consideration venous involvement. It really is a "worldwide research emergency" (Haacke 2010c) because if CCSVI plays a prominent role in the development of multiple sclerosis, treatment will change dramatically to include repair of these venous issues before iron is deposited. The eyes of the MS patients worldwide are focused on MS researchers as they look for well-done research to answer these questions.

This chapter postulates that the hypothesis that MS may be a type of venous insufficiency is reasonable. The next chapter will detail what the Italian research team found when they looked at the hemodynamics of the blood flow in the cerebrospinal systems of MS patients to see if they did have any flow abnormalities. Their groundbreaking findings are nothing short of remarkable.

5

Evidence of Venous Changes in Multiple Sclerosis

It is hard to start a train but harder to stop it—posted on TIMS

Dr. Zamboni wrote the first paper suggesting the theory that MS appeared to have features of a venous disease, as discussed in the last chapter, but detailed research on cerebrospinal hemodynamics did not exist (Zamboni 2006). He needed to do studies on the cerebrospinal hemodynamics to take his theory to the next level.

Dr. Zamboni assembled a team of Italian researchers including both neurology and vascular specialists from Bologna and Ferrara in Italy. His theory that venous pathology accounts for some features of MS posed many questions. The first question that needed an answer was whether people with MS have venous insufficiency in the cerebrospinal system.

They carried out a series of three studies that methodically built one upon the other until they satisfied themselves that they had answered this question. The following review of this groundbreaking research will give the reader a good sense of what, precisely, these researchers evaluated.

Sardinian Children

The Italian research team laid their plans for how to investigate the possibility of altered hemodynamics in people with MS, and as they did this, they wondered if people with known venous problems in their cerebrospinal systems develop MS. The specific question was this: "Might people with jugular problems develop MS over time?"

In fact, Dr. Zamboni himself had studied children with venous abnormalities in Sardinia over 20 years ago (Zamboni 1990). These children had exhibited jugular problems and the research team decided they needed to follow up with those children, now grown, to see if any of these people had developed multiple sclerosis. The researchers were unfortunately not able to locate the entire cohort twenty years later, and so this study is still not published. However, a number of the patients who were located had been diagnosed with MS over the intervening years. This evidence of a previously unknown risk factor was a stunning affirmation that an investigation of the venous model would be critically important.

An Initial Look at Hemodynamics in MS: The First Doppler Study

Because of the lack of research describing the venous hemodynamics of the cerebrospinal system, the researchers had to begin by evaluating the basic issue of how to assess venous blood flow in this complicated area of the body. They chose to use duplex ultrasonography, which is commonly used to evaluate the hemodynamics in other parts of the body, because it is a safe, relatively inexpensive and readily available diagnostic tool. This test gives a real-time view of the actual blood flow in a living person.

Sonography and Reflux

Duplex ultrasonography uses Doppler technology to colorize the blood flow based on which direction it is going. It also gives the operator additional information about the blood vessels themselves with a separate grayscale readout; thus the word *duplex* for two findings in the one Doppler ultrasound test (patients often refer to these tests as simply *Dopplers*). The colorized feature of the diagnostic uses red and blue to differentiate the direction of blood flow. Blood flowing toward the heart is colored blue and should be veins. Blood flowing away from the heart is colored red and should be arteries. If the sonographer is looking at blood flow and it is blue most of the time, signifying a vein, and it periodically turns red for a significant portion of time, then blood flow in that area is refluxing because it is changing direction.

One of the criticisms of vascular ultrasound diagnostics is that they are very dependent on the operator interpretation and settings; it is not "one size fits all." The precise angle that the operator uses with the *transducer* (the device that is pressed against the skin) and the amount of pressure the operator applies greatly affect the reading. Adding to the confusion, some reflux is normal, so the operator has to decide if what they see is something unusual they should record or not. However, in skilled hands with the right training, it gives a valuable assessment of hemodynamics and reliably detects pathologic reverse blood flow (Menegatti and Zamboni 2008).

Recall that blood flow that goes against the physiologic direction is the definition of reflux. Therefore, this colorized way of observing blood flow in a blood vessel is very helpful in determining the existence of reflux that may be indicative of the changes typical of venous insufficiency.

The First Doppler Study Done by the Italian Team

The research team designed their first study to investigate the hemodynamics of MS cerebrospinal systems with 89 MS patients and 60 matched controls (Zamboni et al. 2007). This was an *open-label* observational study, meaning that the person doing the assessment knew the diagnosis of the tested person. The goal was to find a way to evaluate this system using duplex ultrasonography and identify any differences specific to MS patients suggestive of venous insufficiency, as Dr. Zamboni hypothesized in his earlier paper.

Highlights

Highlights of the study were that the deep middle cerebral veins showed reflux in 36 percent of RRMS patients and 42 percent of SPMS patients. However, these evaluations were made through a *transcranial window* (opening between the bones of the head) not previously described and not widely validated in the general medical community, so the data must be considered very preliminary.

The paper states:

> The main finding of our study is the direction of altered hemodynamics just in veins anatomically related to MS lesions, causing a high rate of reverse flow with a chaotic displacement of blood at the activation of the thoracic pump, which is never seen in controls. By contrast in control subjects we assessed a laminar, mono directional outflow, with low velocity, and without reflux, confirming data derived from normal volunteers [Zamboni et al. 2007].

This initial finding supports the possibility that altered venous flow may be common in MS. Further studies were needed to validate the new techniques and findings.

Limitations of the First Study

There were limitations to this initial study. First, it was not blinded. Next, the researchers could not be certain where the blood flow changes were originating from because they did not evaluate the veins outside the head.

And last, they were using an unvalidated approach by evaluating through a newly described transcranial window. These facts demanded further study to validate both the findings and the new approach to evaluation of the deep cerebral veins (Zamboni et al. 2007).

Related Study: Developing the Five-Test Duplex Ultrasonography Protocol

To address this need for wider assessment, Dr. Menegatti and Dr. Zamboni developed and tested a five-test protocol for assessing the complete cerebrospinal system, including extracranial (outside the head — that is, the neck and chest) veins, using duplex ultrasonography. The peer-reviewed journal *Current Neurovascular Research* published the technical methodology (exactly how it was done) (Menegatti and Zamboni 2008).

Later references to *the five-test protocol* in this book refer to the specific sequence of tests using duplex ultrasonography as outlined in Dr. Menegatti and Dr. Zamboni's research. The five-test protocol represents an advancement in technique and interpretation of findings. Using this new technique and diagnostic criteria makes it possible to evaluate the hemodynamics of the cerebrospinal venous system in a new way, although later critics have commented that there is no widely accepted agreement about how to evaluate blood flow in the deep veins of the brain (Krogias et al. 2010), alluding to the unproven status of the techniques.

Looking Deeper into Hemodynamics: Second Study Evaluating MS Patients

The Italian research team carried out a second, more detailed study to evaluate the hemodynamics of the cerebrospinal system in MS patients using the new five-test protocol. This second study was designed to answer the obvious gaps in understanding uncovered in the first study.

Design Details

In this second study, the researchers evaluated cerebrospinal hemodynamics in patients with MS compared to a control group that included people with other types of neurological diseases. There were 109 MS patients and 177 controls (Zamboni et al. 2009d). Unlike the first study, this research was blinded so the doctor doing the sonography and the doctor interpreting the results did not know the diagnosis of the person they were evaluating.

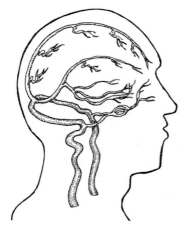

This drawing depicts the major veins of the brain by pretending the brain itself is completely invisible. The superior sagittal sinus curves up over the top of the brain; below it is the inferior sagittal sinus, and below that the deep veins of the brain. The two transverse sinuses are the horizontal sections that lead to the internal jugular veins. The transverse sinuses and everything above them are in the cranium adjacent to brain tissue. The internal jugular veins are the large veins going down the neck and from there the blood drains to the brachiocephalic, the superior vena cava, and finally to the heart to be recirculated. Notice that there is a confluence in the brain where all the veins come together; this confluence allows rerouting. Not shown in this image are the vertebral veins, which drain from the area near the confluence down through the vertebral column in the neck and then into the brachiocephalic. When people are standing, most of the blood from the head drains through the vertebral veins. When lying down the primary route is through the internal jugular veins. When the internal jugular vein is blocked, the blood is rerouted through the vertebral veins in all positions. Image courtesy of Marv Miller.

Results and Discussion from the Work

The researchers did all five of the tests detailed in the five-test protocol on each of the controls and MS patients so that in total they did 1,430 tests. People from the control group only showed problems with blood flow on 24 tests out of the 885 performed on them. People with MS showed problems with abnormal blood flow on 257 tests; only 288 tests were normal among multiple sclerosis patients. Each of these tests is statistically highly significant for MS because the failure rate was so high in MS patients while only the rare control failed.

Nevertheless, what is even more interesting is what happened when they began to analyze the data. They realized no single test was the one that all MS patients failed, but it turned out that in this study all of the MS patients failed at least two and sometimes even more of these tests. None of the controls failed two tests, though a few had failed one (Zamboni et al. 2009d).

This demonstrated a gross overall problem with venous drainage in general in MS patients as compared to controls when they were evaluated using the duplex ultrasonography five-test protocol. It also suggests that a number of locations might be the source of the reflux in the cerebrospinal system and people failed different tests based on the location of the stenosis and type of reflux they individually manifested.

The researchers concluded that this combination of tests could be useful as a diagnostic for multiple sclerosis because patients with MS showed many changes in hemodynamics in comparison to healthy people. However, they mentioned that there is a need for training and assessment of the ability of other technicians to do these newly described duplex ultrasonography tests (Zamboni et al. 2009d).

Third Doppler Study Evaluating MS: The Addition of Venograms

To further investigate and confirm the findings, the research team designed a third study. They designed this study to use the five-test protocol, but, importantly, this study also included venograms to prove that actual physical alterations in the veins caused the altered hemodynamics seen in people with MS.

After deliberation, the Ethics Committee of the Ferrara University Hospital finally approved of performing venograms on the MS patients who showed the two abnormal findings parameter of the five-test protocol (Zamboni et al. 2009c). A venogram is an invasive test that has some risk; therefore venograms were only justifiable once there was reasonable evidence that there was a problem with venous drainage in people with MS. Fortunately, the findings of the earlier studies supported the use of venograms. The addition of venograms would give the researchers a much fuller, more objective picture of the venous hemodynamics in MS patients and would confirm the five-test protocol as a valuable diagnostic.

Study Design and Recruitment

The third study included 65 patients with MS and 235 controls. Controls included people with cardiovascular disease, other neurological disease, and 48 people already scheduled for venograms with other kinds of vascular disease. The researchers would check the cerebrospinal system of patients getting venograms for these other vascular issues to see if they had CCSVI or occlusions (Zamboni et al. 2009c).

The patients with MS showed hemodynamic abnormalities using the five-test protocol exactly as in the second study. As in the previous work, blinded researchers identified MS patients by looking for people demonstrating two abnormal findings (Zamboni et al. 2009c).

Similar to the previous study, the number of normal tests in the 235 non–MS controls was 1,142, whereas only 33 tests were abnormal (remember, each patient received 5 tests). In the 65 MS patients, there were only 145 normal tests while the abnormal tests numbered higher at 180. This constitutes a 42-fold increase in abnormal findings in the MS group (Zamboni et al. 2009c). With the completion of the five-test protocol examinations, the blinded part of this study was done. The second stage of this study included venograms; this part of the study was not blinded.

Venograms Explained

Venograms are an invasive kind of diagnostic. In order to do a venogram on a vein, the blood vessel is accessed through a small hole in the skin; then the physician threads a small catheter through the venous system. The physician manipulates the steerable catheter until it gets to the area he wants to evaluate and/or treat. Once the catheter is in the correct location, he injects dye through it and observes how the dye flows through the blood vessels. To see this he uses a machine called a fluoroscope.

A fluoroscope is very similar to an X-ray, although it creates real-time pictures that make a kind of X-ray movie. With this device the dye can be observed as it moves through the blood vessel, and any strictures, blockages, occlusions or other abnormalities can also be seen. The physician is additionally able to visualize churning and chaotic blood flow or reflux.

Collateral circulation, which is a physiological response to reflux (as was discussed in chapter 4), is also visible using the venogram. The presence of collateral circulation is an additional confirmation of a significant occlusion in the vein. Though it was not done in Dr. Zamboni's third study, if the physician needs more information he can introduce a small ultrasound device through the catheter to take readings inside the vein. This intravascular ultrasound (IVUS) generates more information about abnormalities seen in the vein. The physician can also repair abnormalities identified during the venogram by introducing small medical instruments, such as angioplasty balloons, through the same catheter that introduces the dye.

Venograms give a more detailed visualization of the actual blood vessels than the five-test protocol, which looks specifically at blood flow. The addition of findings from venograms was the perfect way to build upon the ultrasound work done in the first half of this study and in the earlier two studies. Venograms were also a way to confirm that the five-test protocol was a valid diagnostic because they are less subject to operator interpretation than ultrasound and are widely considered the gold standard for diagnosis of vascular abnormalities (Lensing et al. 1992).

Study Venograms

After completing the blinded first half of the study in which the Italian researchers examined people with the five-test protocol using duplex ultra-

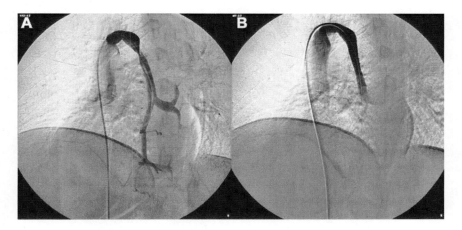

In this image, venography shows a dramatic twisting of the azygous vein just below the arch with reflux toward the spine and (B) endovascular correction by stent insertion and reflux disappearance. Image and caption originally published in "A Prospective Open-Label Study of Endovascular Treatment of Chronic Cerebrospinal Venous Insufficiency" (Zamboni et al. 2009b). Used with permission. The azygous vein is in the chest and, when occluded, blood reroutes through the spinal system.

sonography, they performed the second half of the study using venograms. The physicians were not blinded when doing the venograms. What the researchers discovered was that all the MS patients had some type of stenosis of the cerebrospinal system. None of the control persons had stenoses (Zamboni et al. 2009c).

In the MS patients, they saw actual twisted veins, flaps in the veins, inverted valves, stenosis or narrowed areas, atresia and otherwise altered or malformed veins. These anomalies were clearly the cause of the reflux and failures on the five-test protocol. This confirmed the finding that two abnormal readings on the protocol they had designed correlated with actual physical abnormalities in the veins (Zamboni et al. 2009c).

Researchers characterized the tissue removed from the vein as having an embryological origin (Lee et al. 2010). This was later identified as a venous truncular malformation (Lee et al. 2009), which will be discussed in detail later in this book.

Pressure Differences

The research team evaluated the pressure difference across the occluded areas inside the veins. In MS patients with stenoses, the readings inside the vein on the brain's side of the blockage were higher than they were on the other side. In the example cited in the research paper, the pressure difference across the azygous was 3.9 cm higher on the up stream of the occlusion (Zamboni et al. 2009c). The researchers considered this amount of pressure difference significant because this is a low-pressure system and readings in this range represent treatable stenoses, as established by other researchers (Labropoulos et al. 2007).

An important finding in this study was that there appears to be no difference in terms of the presence or absence of venous malformations when comparing patients treated with immune-modulating or -suppressing drugs and those not treated.

> If vessel abnormalities were due to an inflammatory-autoimmune disease, they would be less frequent in patients treated with immunomodulating/immuno-suppressant agents. On the contrary, our analysis in the RR-SP group did not demonstrate an increased number of extracranial venous stenosing lesions in untreated as compared to treated patients [Zamboni et al. 2009c].

This suggests that the stenoses are not an inflammatory reaction caused by the MS process.

PPMS Is Special

What this research team did notice was a pattern of stenosis correlated with PPMS, suggesting that perhaps the specific area that has altered hemodynamics influences this type of MS (Zamboni et al. 2009c). The number of patients seen in this research was small, though (only 10 people had PPMS), so cautious interpretation is necessary. Replication by other researchers on larger numbers of patients will clarify this phenomenon.

Summary: The Ferrara and Bologna Team's Research

The Italian research team evaluated a total 735 people in this series of three studies:

Study 1: 89 MS patients and 60 matched controls.
Study 2: 109 MS patients and 177 controls (blinded).
Study 3: 65 MS patients and 235 controls (blinded, with venograms).

Dr. Zamboni and the team at Ferrara and Bologna offered a cogent and well-supported set of peer-reviewed research papers. This series of studies has made a very compelling case for the possibility that multiple sclerosis has a significant venous component, starting with the hypothesis detailed in "The Big Idea" and concluding with the third Doppler study that included venograms. Taken together with the research cited in earlier chapters, in particular the extensive historical evidence for a vascular component in MS, the support for this hypothesis is much better than the typical new hypothesis of MS causation.

However, the scientific community must consider this research preliminary until other teams of workers replicate the findings in blinded studies. Unfortunately, replication has not proven to be simple. The most significant obstacle to replication is that duplex ultrasonography in the cerebrospinal system as done by the Italian researchers is very difficult for other researchers and physicians to perform. Doppler exams are always operator-dependent but in addition these particular techniques and the way the Italian research team identified the problems in the deep veins are new, and together this means reliable results are very difficult to achieve, even for experts in the field of sonography (Dake 2010b).

Related Study: Untrained Sonographers

MS patients around the world hearing about the Zamboni research were interested in seeking assessment in their local communities. Patients seeking these evaluations reported on the Internet that local sonographers were unable to see anything that they considered unusual, even if they had read the Menegatti and Zamboni 2008 paper and were trying to replicate the five-test protocol. Dr. Menegatti undertook a study to evaluate how well sonographers with no specialized training were able to perform these advanced colorized duplex Doppler tests (Menegatti et al. 2010).

The researchers designed the study so that both sonographers specially trained in detecting altered cerebrospinal venous hemodynamics with the five-test protocol and sonographers without this special training would test people with MS. The test results of the two skill levels were compared to see what impact training had on diagnostic findings.

This study revealed that trained people produced test results that were in agreement with one another; the findings of one trained sonographer were the same as another's on the same patient. However, sonographers who had not had training were unable to generate consistent findings (Menegatti et al. 2010).

Valsalva Pitfalls

In all of Dr. Zamboni's research, the "Valsalva" maneuver when performing assessment using the five-test protocol was specifically avoided. This is important because cerebral Doppler exams that use the Valsalva are common and evaluate for problems with jugular valve competence unrelated to CCSVI.

Most people have a valve at the bottom of the internal jugular vein. This valve prevents blood from refluxing up into the brain when a person has an increase in pressure in the chest. A strong cough or the Valsalva maneuver, which is when someone holds their breath and then "pushes" as if to have a bowel movement, causes temporary reflux from the chest through the jugular toward the brain if the valve does not work correctly. People with transient global amnesia and 25 percent of healthy people have this problem with an incompetent jugular valve (Cejas et al. 2010).

Evaluating the competence of the jugular valves using the Valsalva maneuver is not the same as the five-test protocol. The five-test protocol evaluates to see if stenosis obstructs venous blood flow so that the blood cannot drain from the cerebrospinal system and there is venous insufficiency. Jugular valve incompetence causes transient reflux when there is a sudden increase in thoracic pressure. This temporary problem is unrelated to ongoing reflux caused by venous outflow obstruction. Other research teams attempting to replicate the Italian research using Dopplers have sometimes used the more familiar Valsalva test for valve competency (Doepp et al. 2010).

Dr. Zamboni is very restrained when interviewed about his research. He carefully points out the facts and the evidence that he has been building in the literature since 2006 (Favaro 2009). He will admit that personally he believes CCSVI is a significant part of the pathology of MS, but he does not say that MS is not autoimmune nor does he make any inflated claims of "cure." Dr. Zamboni says other researchers need to do similar work to confirm his findings and build upon the research to elucidate the full scope of this issue.

Fortunately, other researchers have accepted this challenge and have begun replicating research. The next section discusses the efforts of other researchers to evaluate people with MS for altered blood flow.

Peer Commentary and Support

Work by the Italian research team strongly suggests that people with multiple sclerosis specifically have venous malformations in the cerebrospinal system. The rest of the research community has begun to add to the body of knowledge by doing their own research.

The first reviews on this groundbreaking research came in the form of referenced comments made by other physicians reading the research in the *Journal of Neurology, Neurosurgery and Psychiatry* in response to the paper published in December 2008 titled "Chronic Cerebrospinal Venous Insufficiency in Patients with Multiple Sclerosis." This was the third color Doppler study that included venograms (discussed previously). When this paper was published, it really generated a buzz.

Marian Simka, MD, a vascular surgeon, offered a well-referenced comment in a letter to the editor titled "Chronic Cerebrospinal Venous Insufficiency: A Potential Weakening Factor in the Blood Brain Barrier" (Simka 2009d), which supported the idea that perhaps this venous hemodynamic could trigger MS autoimmune activation. He described how alterations in shear stress may impair the blood-brain barrier.

In his comment, Steven Brenner, MD, an American neurologist, focused on the fact that MS researchers have long known the perivenous nature of the plaques in MS. He then offered that the alterations in hemodynamics seen by Zamboni might result in breakdown of the BBB, then a secondary exposure of central nervous system antigens to the peripheral immune system. He speculated this could be the cause of autoimmunity (Brenner 2009).

Claude Francesci, a French vascular surgeon, commented that the assigned name of "chronic cerebrospinal venous insufficiency" correctly defines the changes Dr. Zamboni documents in MS patients' vascular systems. This is extremely important affirmation of how specialists in the vascular field view the conclusions drawn by Dr. Zamboni.

Dr. Francesci also made an important point regarding collateral circles, commenting that when the venous outflow is deviated to a shunt it becomes very slow circulation because it is operating under the effects of *distal cardiac residual pressure* (a long way from the heart, not much pressure) and the thoracic pump. He postulated that the anomaly of shunted blood is connected to slow mean transit time documented previously in the brains of people with MS (Francesci 2009).

In addition to these positive comments, the Zamboni paper was cited by Pirko and Zivadinov in their comment published in *Neurology* titled "Transcranial Sonography of Deep Gray Nuclei: A New Outcome Measure in Multiple Sclerosis?" (Pirko and Zivadinov 2009). They were commenting on a paper titled "Transcranial Brain Sonography Findings Predict Disease Progression in Multiple Sclerosis." The conclusion mentioned on the abstract of that paper states, "Neurodegenerative disease-like deep gray matter lesions can be frequently detected by transcranial sonography (TCS) in patients with multiple sclerosis (MS). Findings suggest that TCS shows changes of brain iron metabolism which correlate with future progress of MS" (Walter et al. 2009).

In a research paper out of Australia in January 2010 researchers comment, "The clinical features and MRI characteristics of the medullary lesions suggest an impairment of venous drainage. We propose that the formation of these wedge-shaped lesions may be related to the pattern of venous drainage in the ventral medulla and raised venous pressure due to chronic cerebrospinal venous insufficiency which has recently been described in MS" (Qui et al. 2010).

According to another recent study, patients with multiple sclerosis who also have other vascular diseases appear to have a worse prognosis than people who do not. Researchers showed that patients with the comorbidity of MS and a vascular disease progressed faster and experienced worse MS outcomes (Marrie et al. 2010).

A recent published review of chronic cerebrospinal venous insufficiency done by Ashton Embry, PhD, of Direct-MS, the second-largest charity in Canada advocating for multiple sclerosis patients, puts forth the hypothesis that MS is an autoimmune disease and that the presence of CCSVI worsens it: "The final intriguing result is that the higher the disability the higher the chance that CCSVI is involved. Given the congenital origin of the vascular malformations, such a result indicates that CCSVI is an adjuvant to the MS process. This means if one has MS and CCSVI they have a much higher chance of progressing to a higher disability level" (Embry 2010a).

The recognition of the Zamboni research both by positive comments on the paradigm and the use of the work in citation to discuss other medical literature among peers shows how important this work is in the medical community. This is an auspicious beginning for this new model.

Replication: Supporting Studies

Scientific rigor demands that other people be able to replicate research to duplicate the findings and prove that what the original research team reported is valid. This section discusses new research supporting the Zamboni model.

Marian Simka, MD, Euromedic, Department of Vascular and Endovascular Surgery in Katowice

Dr. Simka read the third study including venograms and was inspired to take the time to research and publish the previously mentioned a comment. He then decided to undertake a study to replicate the Italian team's research. In his small study, Dr. Simka tested 8 patients with multiple sclerosis and confirmed the Zamboni findings; all patients showed more than 2 abnormal findings with the five-test protocol. This work was not blinded or controlled (Simka et al. 2009).

Dr. Simka states he found it much more difficult than expected to assess the intracranial hemodynamics with duplex ultrasound. He said there was a significant learning curve and it took his team weeks to complete the observational study (Marian Simka, MD, personal communication, May 30, 2010).

Following the initial study, Dr. Simka led a team of researchers in a larger study. This open-label study assessed 70 people with MS using the Zamboni duplex ultrasound five-test protocol. They discovered that 90 percent of these people showed two abnormal findings. The kinds of actual physical problems that they were able to see with this limited technology (as opposed to venograms) were inverted valves and abnormal membranes that blocked the blood flow. These were most often at the place where the internal jugular vein and brachiocephalic vein met and were observed in 58 percent of the patients (Simka et al. 2010c).

Dr. Simka has commented that he now looks at the jugulars in people who need color Doppler exams of their carotid arteries. He does see some seemingly healthy people who do not have MS but who fit the two abnormal findings parameter. Dr. Simka is not the only researcher outside of the Italian research to see two abnormal findings in some supposedly normal people (Zivadinov 2010). This suggests as researchers evaluate larger numbers of people in other centers, it may prove to be true that the two abnormal tests parameter is not exclusive to people with MS.

Dr. Simka has since gone on to a private clinic and is now doing an approved study including angioplasty or stent treatment of stenosis in patients with MS and CCSVI. This next phase of research includes venograms and treatment. He has commented that in his team's view further studies to see if people with MS have altered hemodynamics would be wasting time. They feel the more pressing challenge is determining how to reliably evaluate and treat these issues (Marian Simka, MD, personal communication, May 30, 2010).

King Abdullah University Hospital, Jordan University of Science and Technology, Jordan

Dr. Al-Omari and Dr. Rousan replicated the Zamboni Doppler work on 25 patients with MS and 25 controls. 92 percent of MS patients showed abnormal findings with 84 percent of them meeting the criteria for CCSVI. 24 percent of controls had abnormal findings, but none of them met the criteria for CCSVI. These researchers concluded that hemodynamic abnormalities involving the internal jugular vein are strongly associated with multiple sclerosis (Al-Omari and Rousan 2010).

Buffalo Neuroimaging Analysis Center
in Buffalo, New York

Jacobs Neurological Institute (JNI) and its associated Buffalo Neuroimaging Analysis Center (BNAC) in Buffalo, New York, an affiliate of SUNY, followed several of Dr. Zamboni's patients with their 3 Tesla MRI. The research team in Ferrara and Bologna has been working with researchers from JNI/BNAC in an international collaboration that has resulted in many interesting papers on this new paradigm, several of which are described below.

VHISS AND CSF FLOW DYNAMICS • Researchers at BNAC developed a way to grade the findings from a person's colorized Doppler study to quantify the severity of cerebrospinal venous insufficiency in an individual. This new assessment tool is called the cerebral venous hemodynamics insufficiency severity score (VHISS). Similar to the EDSS, it provides a tool to assign a number so that physicians may grade the severity of venous insufficiency in individual patients.

Using this new scoring system, the team at BNAC was able to compare severity of reduced venous hemodynamics in 16 MS patients to that of eight normal controls. After evaluating the blood flow of each individual person, the researchers evaluated the cerebrospinal fluid (CSF) dynamics as well.

The results of the study showed that more severe venous insufficiency was highly correlated with impaired CSF flow dynamics. This means that if a patient's blood flow was refluxing, the fluid in their brain was not flowing correctly either. This suggests that impaired blood flow correlates with flow problems in the cerebrospinal fluid (Zamboni et al. 2009e). Dr. Zamboni has published an editorial in which he suggests that the reason for this is that the increase in venous pressure, even though modest, reduces the resorption of the cerebrospinal fluid (Zamboni 2010).

Brain atrophy is related to reduced resorbtion of cerebrospinal fluid in patients with idiopathic normal pressure hydrocephalus as well (Bradley 2008). It may be that atrophy in MS patients is related to this problem with cerebrospinal fluid dynamics. The findings from this work led to the study discussed in the next section.

VENOUS HEMODYNAMICS AND ATROPHY • The study mentioned above looked at cerebrospinal flow and compared it to venous hemodynamics, but the same team also did a related study to compare venous hemodynamics (VH) to the loss of brain volume (atrophy) in association with altered cerebrospinal fluid flow. The researchers evaluated patients using the Doppler examinations to assess their hemodynamics, and then performed an MRI to assess the loss of brain volume and cerebrospinal fluid flow. The conclusion was that more

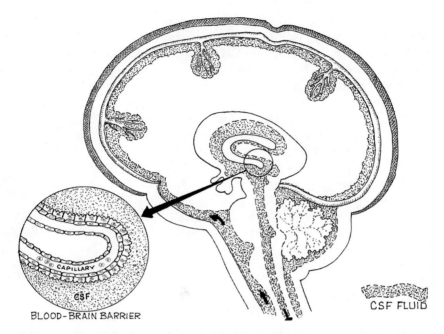

This image shows how the cerebrospinal fluid bathes the brain. The fluid is made in the choroid plexus in the middle of the brain and is resorbed via the veins through the BBB. Ordinarily this cycle of creation and resorbtions results in four exchanges of CSF in a day. Congestion, and thus mildly increased pressure, of the veins may theoretically hamper resorbtion. Image courtesy of Marv Miller.

severely altered hemodynamics was associated with poorer flow in the cerebrospinal fluid and atrophy of the brain. The conclusion states: "The number of anomalous VH criteria were measured using an echo-color Doppler, whereas CSF flow, atrophy and lesion measures were obtained from quantitative magnetic resonance imaging (MRI)s.... CONCLUSION: VH changes occur more frequently in MS patients than controls. Altered VH is associated with abnormal CSF flow dynamics and decreased brain volume" (Zamboni et al. 2010). This suggests that not only do these changes in the venous hemodynamics result in changes in the CSF, but that these changes are also associated with decreased brain volume. This is important because decreased brain volume is a change that radiologists note in people when MS becomes progressive. The association of atrophy with the severity of altered venous hemodynamics is an important finding that will require more research for better understanding of what this association means.

VENOUS HEMODYNAMICS AND IRON DEPOSITS • Another study assessed flow dynamics in 16 MS patients and 8 matched controls to see if they could establish any correlation between venous hemodynamics and iron deposits. This study found that none of the healthy controls had issues with CCSVI but all the MS patients had problems with VH that qualified them as having CCSVI. Iron deposits in the deep brain were highly correlated with the blood flow problems (Zivadinov et al. 2010).

LARGE DOPPLER STUDY • Drs. Bianca Weinstock-Guttman and Robert Zivadinov, both at JNI, have begun an astonishingly large study using the duplex ultrasonography five-test protocol to assess a projected 1,500 MS patients and controls for CCSVI. The trial is named the Combined Transcranial and Extracranial Venous Doppler Evaluation in Multiple Sclerosis and Related Diseases (the CTEVD study). The researchers designed the study to take place in three phases with results released after each phase over two years.

Dr. Zivadinov reviewed the phase 1 results at the American Academy of Neurology and NMSS open forum in Toronto on April 14, 2010. The assessment team used Dr. Zamboni's protocol to evaluate the first 499 people. They had technical difficulty performing the second test of the protocol, and because of this, their results are quite different from Dr. Zamboni's.

The second test in Dr. Menegatti and Dr. Zamboni's protocol evaluates the deep cerebral veins. In the Italian research, 61 percent of MS patients had an abnormal reading in this test as one of their "two abnormal tests." Because the CTEVD study was unable to perform this test in one third of their patients, the researchers calculated the totals of MS patients differently and there is a group of patients called "borderline." These borderline people had one abnormal test that might have met the "two abnormal tests" parameter if the missing test had been done.

The percentage of patients with MS who showed CCSVI on the five-test protocol was 56 percent, not counting the borderline patients. If the borderline people are included, the percentage rises to 62 percent. The number of controls with CCSVI was 22 percent without the borderline, and 25 percent with the borderline included (Zivadinov 2010).

Another analysis performed by the researchers in this CTEVD study was how often people failed an individual test. They found that the test most often failed by people with MS was test number three, which looks at the vein and evaluates the blood vessel itself. They most often saw flaps, membranes, and abnormalities inside the vein in patients with secondary progressive MS. SPMS patients had a 90 percent prevalence of this problem in this research (Zivadinov 2010).

Dr. Zivadinov commented on this study and the discrepancy between his work and Dr. Zamboni's. He stated in an interview that differences in equipment and technique may account for the discordant findings (Zivadinov

2010). The next two phases of this large Doppler study will further clarify this issue.

Note that even with MS patients showing CCSVI 56 percent of the time and controls showing this issue 25 percent of the time, this is similar to the HLA genetic risk factor for MS (Zivadinov 2010). Additionally, other research suggests that having both MS and a vascular disease worsens the prognosis for the MS patient (Marrie et al. 2010).

PATTERNS OF STENOSIS • The Ferrara and Bologna research team reported in their study with venograms that there were 4 patterns of stenosis seen (Zamboni et al. 2009c). In a follow-up study done by researchers in Italy, they discovered that these patterns were associated with different disease types; for example, a pattern they labeled type D was more common in patients with spinal cord lesions. In type D, the azygous system was affected, sometimes in several areas, so that the blood refluxed through the intra-spinal veins back to the vertebral veins and up into the deep cerebral veins to seek a way out through the internal jugular veins. This suggests that the location of the stenosis may account for the fact that MS presents differently with some PPMS patients and some RRMS (Bartolomei et al. 2010).

CHRONIC FATIGUE IN MS AND RELATION TO CCSVI • A research team comprised of some members of Dr. Zamboni's original team and new researchers evaluated how treatment of CCSVI influenced fatigue as measured by the Fatigue Severity Scale (FSS) and Modified Fatigue Impact Scale (MFIS). This research revealed a dramatic reduction in fatigue in treated people, suggesting that fatigue may be the symptom of CCSVI (Malagoni et al. 2010). This might suggest that fatigue is caused by CCSVI and may be separate from symptoms of MS.

DOPPLER ULTRASOUND VERSUS MRV • Researchers from BNAC and Italy designed a study to test magnetic resonance venography (MRV) in comparison to both the five-test protocol administered by trained people and venograms for diagnosing CCSVI in multiple sclerosis patients. Healthy controls in this study did not receive venograms, though they did receive the five-test protocol and MRV. The result was that the five-test protocol once again identified CCSVI in all MS patients but healthy controls showed normal blood flow. Venograms confirmed CCSVI in all MS patients.

Then the researchers looked at the MRV findings and discovered this diagnostic had only about 55 percent accuracy (average of two types tested) for identifying venous changes related to CCSVI. By contrast, the five-test ultrasound protocol administered by trained people demonstrated accuracy of 95 percent (Hojnacki et al. 2010).

This highlights one of the brewing controversies inside the field of study in CCSVI. Dr. Zamboni continues to be committed to the value of duplex ultrasound. He is adamant that CCSVI comprises a problem in blood flow in very specific areas of the brain and not simply stenoses or blockages. He believes duplex ultrasound is the best method for evaluating blood flow. Other researchers, such as Dr. Haacke (mentioned section after next), are working to refine a less operator-dependent evaluation using MRV and SWI MRI. This will likely continue to be an area of active research and debate until everyone agrees there is a clearly superior method for reliable evaluation and diagnosis of CCSVI.

Interventional Radiologists in Kuwait

In Kuwait the government has approved of both assessment and treatment for their citizens. The research there involves a collaborative effort between neurology and vascular doctors, a model for the future.

Interventional radiologists in Kuwait have reported that they carried out testing on 100 patients to evaluate for CCSVI in multiple sclerosis. In this study, MS patients showed signs of CCSVI with colorized Dopplers 81 percent of the time and with MRV 96 percent of the time. Healthy controls showed an abnormal Doppler test 7 percent of the time. The research team in Kuwait intends to treat these patients and follow them at 3, 6, 9, and 12 months with repeat colorized Doppler exams, MRI scans and neurological testing to see how treatment impacts MS. Interested people can follow this work at www.ccsvikuwait.com.

E. Mark Haacke, PhD, and SWI MRI: Information for Radiologists by Dr. Haacke

Susceptibility weighted imaging is a newer MRI technique often referred to as SWI MRI, or more commonly as just SWI. It is a special way of processing gradient echo imaging data to provide different assessments of the brain that allows the radiologist to see small veins in the brain with unprecedented detail as well as iron deposits.

This new technique has been created and studied in peer-reviewed research by E. Mark Haacke, PhD, a physicist, who has been working this approach since 1997 at the MRI Institute for Biomedical Research and Wayne State University in Michigan. Currently, SWI is offered only by machines made by Siemens Healthcare, but the data itself can be collected on other manufacturers' systems and processed with special software developed by Dr. Haacke's group called SPIN (signal processing in nuclear magnetic resonance).

SWI has proven valuable for imaging not only multiple sclerosis but also aging, Parkinson's disease, stroke and traumatic brain injury.

SWI works on the principle that iron in the body can be used as an intrinsic contrast agent. A contrast agent often used for MS patients is gadolinium, which allows the MRI to see any areas where there is active inflammation. In SWI, iron in the form of ferritin, hemosiderin, or deoxyhemoglobin can be quantified by SPIN to highlight abnormalities often not seen with conventional MRI. This technology uses the iron as a contrast agent.

The data generated by SWI has bearing on the debate about CCSVI because it is able to image very small veins, oxygen saturation and iron in tissue. In MS, pathological iron deposits are extensive and associated with disability, while inflammatory lesions in the white matter are less correlated with disability (Bakshi et al. 2002; Zhang et al. 2007a; Neema et al. 2009).

Dr. Haacke has documented the fact that even at a young age iron deposits are higher in MS patients than in controls. This mirrors the fact that there is extensive loss of NAA (n-acetyle aspartate), showing that there is axonal damage in the brains of patients early in the disease (Filippi et al. 2003). The iron deposits are especially noticeable in the basal ganglia and thalamus, areas in the gray matter of the brain. Iron is also noted in lesions and as rings around some lesions. By comparing SWI MRI to autopsy samples, researchers have demonstrated that iron seen in these structures mimics iron seen with other techniques. Because this is still an experimental way of evaluating MS, this confirmation is an important step leading to eventual acceptance of the technology. This iron seen in the brain is thought to be in the form of hemosiderin, which brings the work full circle back to Dr. Zamboni's "big idea" paper discussed in chapter 4 because hemosiderin is thought to be related to extravasated red blood cells, as opposed to ferritin, which is simply the body's way of storing out-of-place iron.

Another issue that may be evaluated with this technology is oxygen levels in the blood. When blood goes through the capillary bed (chapter 4), it surrenders oxygen and then needs to go through the venous system back to the heart and lungs to re-oxygenate. Dr. Yulin Ge (Ge et al. 2009) has shown that SWI is able to detect the fact that the veins are less conspicuous in MS patients, which suggests there is not as much deoxyhemoglobin in their blood. This could imply tissue that is not fully extracting the oxygen or it could be the result of a reduced venous blood volume locally. Both are suggestive that the tissue may be ischemic (suffering from a lack of oxygen). If the tissue is without oxygen for long enough, it becomes necrotic (it dies).

The reason this is an issue is that SWI is another way to confirm or deny that the vascular changes the Ferrara team documented match up with facts determined by using this new technology. Because this approach is less open to interpretation and operator skill than the colorized Doppler exams using the five-test protocol, it may be a means to complement the other ongoing research to prove or disprove the new CCSVI theory; many centers could use the SWI and the results would be consistent and reliable.

In theory, the SWI concept can be used in all manufacturers' systems but the data will need to be processed using SPIN. This means multiple interested facilities can be recruited to do these particular SWI assessments on a large number of MS patients, quickly affirming or denying the role of iron and its correlation with the CCSVI paradigm.

Another evaluation that can be performed using MRI/MRV is flow quantification — essentially checking the blood flow with magnetic resonance technology instead of ultrasound. Flow quantification evaluates the blood flow in the cerebrospinal system and can be carried out during the same exam that includes SWI, though the complete test including SWI MRI, standard MRI, MRV and flow quantification takes longer. The advantage is that unlike duplex ultrasonography, this is an objective test that is not operator-dependent, yet it still evaluates blood flow in the cerebrospinal system. MRI is more expensive than Doppler ultrasound but also more extensive and more complete as well.

Dr. Haacke is actively recruiting centers around the world to carry out these assessments. These centers of excellence will generate data under the guidance of an IRB trial.

A new study by Dr. Haacke looking at iron deposits with SWI in MS patients revealed that not only do patients with MS have more iron in their basal ganglia and thalamus than normal people, but the iron accumulates backward along the vein as well (Haacke et al. 2010). This supports the idea that a countercurrent refluxing blood flow causes iron deposits in MS. In chronic venous disease, iron and damage accumulate backward along the refluxing vein (Zamboni 2006). To date, much of Dr. Haacke's findings are potentially supportive of Dr. Zamboni's theory.

The effort currently under way at the MRI institute is to recruit facilities all over the world to do the specific MRI protocol. This protocol images the veins in the head and neck and quantifies blood flow and evaluates iron in MS brain tissue using SWI. Researchers will also refine the protocol as the body of knowledge grows so that the imaging protocol and interpretation of the data will improve. This will contribute immeasurably to the body of knowledge about CCSVI. Dr. Haacke plans to pool the data so that MS patients can be more completely analyzed and researchers can review the data for specific venous abnormalities (E. Mark Haacke, PhD, personal communication, April 20, 2010).

The first two centers using this thorough protocol are the False Creek Imaging Center (BC, Canada) and the Hubbard Foundation (San Diego, USA) (see chapters 6 and 8). However, the latter currently has an approved IRB and they will utilize Dr. Haacke's protocol for magnetic resonance evaluation of CCSVI. The former also hopes to participate in the IRB in the near future.

These "centers of excellence" will offer state-of-the-art advanced diagnostics for the MS patient seeking evaluation and will ensure that data obtained from the diagnostics contributes in a meaningful way to understanding of CCSVI. For radiologists interested in being involved in this project, the current reproducible protocol can be found at www.ms-mri.com and can be downloaded easily and run on systems that are preferably 1.5T or 3T or higher in field strength.

Other Supportive Work: Franz Schelling, MD

Franz Schelling, MD, a physician from Austria, began looking at venous disease as a potential cause of multiple sclerosis in the early 1980s. Dr. Schelling did an in-depth review of the entire body of MS literature beginning in the 1880s and discovered that venous connections had been known and documented from the earliest days, but were systematically ignored (Schelling 2004). Dr. Schelling's work was not taken seriously until recently, when the discoveries made by Dr. Zamboni and the subsequent replication made it clear that Dr. Schelling was ahead of the curve in recognizing that something important had been missed regarding the blood flow in patients with multiple sclerosis.

The International Union of Phlebology

The International Union of Phlebology (IUP) is an international group that sets policy and makes consensus decisions about issues affecting the field. *Phlebology* is the European word for study of vascular issues. In 2009, the team at Ferrara sent tissue samples removed from MS patients to Dr. Gabbiani in Switzerland. These samples were tested and the findings presented at the IUP conference in December 2009.

The consensus of the attending 48 experts in the field regarding the findings was unanimous: the tissue samples removed from MS patients in blocking areas should be classified as truncular venous malformations. This means the tissue that developed into a blockage of some type was likely present from birth.

In related research Dr. Lee explains how embryologic tissue becomes a venous malformation. Embryos have blood vessels that babies and adults do not have. These embryological vessels have to be removed and/or remodeled by the body as the embryo develops in the womb. In some cases, the primitive vessels will no longer be needed and they will shrink away; in other cases they grow, or attach to another vessel and eventually become part of adult circulation. When a remnant of this embryological vascular tissue does not remodel as it should and leaves a malformed area, it can cause problems with circulation. This kind of embryological tissue causes venous truncular malformations like Budd-Chiari syndrome. Embryological tissue can be positively identified in the lab (Lee et al. 2010).

Dr. Lee makes the comment that it is a very simple membranous web in the hepatic venous system of a Budd-Chiari patient that causes portal hypertension and profound damage to the liver. "A similar condition involving the head and neck venous system may cause chronic cerebrospinal venous insufficiency (CCSVI) and may be involved in development or exacerbation of multiple sclerosis" (Lee et al. 2010).

Contradicting Research

As more researchers evaluate the cerebrospinal venous hemodynamics in people with MS, some results contradict the initial findings. This is typical in science as physicians begin to understand and define this phenomenon.

Counter CCSVI Studies

A study that evaluated 56 people with MS and 20 healthy controls using a variety of Doppler ultrasound techniques found normal blood flow in all subjects, with the exception of one person. The researchers attempted to replicate the five-test protocol as described by Menegatti and Zamboni as well as doing an additional test to check for jugular valve incompetence using the Valsalva maneuver and evaluating blood volume flow.

The authors attributed the striking difference between this study and Dr. Zamboni's studies to different techniques. They felt the addition of the Valsalva maneuver to assess for jugular valve competence was an important addition to their methodology that disputes Dr. Zamboni's approach. The reason is, they suggest, that incompetency of the valve could cause reflux that would confuse the clinical picture. In the discussion, they mentioned numerous ways in which an improper technique might suggest reflux and stenosis when none exists (Doepp et al. 2010).

The study authors did not mention the fact that actual stenosis was found with venograms in Dr. Zamboni's third study; their arguments focused on the Doppler methodology.

Another group of MS researchers in Germany reviewed Dr. Zamboni's research and argued strongly against it on several grounds:

First concerning the validity of published data, second with regard to the plausibility in view of the currently approved pathogenetic model of MS, and third with regard to the compatibility with preliminary neurosonological findings in a small but unselected cohort of patients at our department. The authors conclude that the "chronic cerebrospinal venous insufficiency (CCSVI)" cannot represent the exclusive pathogenetic factor in the pathogenesis of MS. In our cohort, only 20 percent of the patients fulfilled the required neurosonological features of CCSVI [Krogias et al. 2010].

They also point out that "there is no agreement in the doppler literature about how to define veins draining from the ventricular planes towards the cortical or subcortical gray matter" (Krogias et al. 2010). They are arguing that there are no established criteria, so no one can say whether the Italian research is looking at something of real clinical significance when evaluating this deep vein hemodynamic in the brain. The authors go on to state that CCSVI and its hypothesis are speculative and patients with MS should not consider treatment.

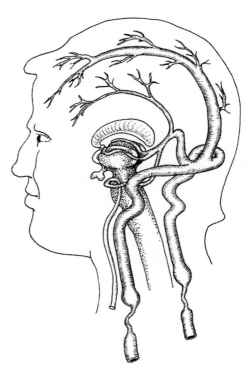

Published Opinion Against the CCSVI Concept

A group of prominent MS neurologists/researchers documented their opinion regarding the CCSVI theory. They make many substantive points. One is that other researchers have not investigated the intracranial venous return prior to this time and therefore there is a lack of established standards with which to compare Dr.

This drawing depicts the veins of the brain in relation to the brain stem and the thalamus. The brain itself is invisible. Dr. Haacke's work with SWI shows iron buildup in the area near the top of the brain stem called the pulvinar thalamus. The internal jugular veins are shown with stenosis. Image courtesy of Marv Miller.

Zamboni's findings (Khan et al. 2010). They are arguing that stenosed veins may be normal.

They also offer several counteropinions based on epidemiology. They point out that MS is "autoimmune in nature with complex T and B cell responses" (Khan et al. 2010) and that nearly two-thirds of MS patients are women, strengthening their argument by mentioning that other autoimmune diseases are more common in women. They further propose that if MS were a vascular phenomenon it should become more common as people got older, yet MS is rarely diagnosed after the age of 50. In addition, they mention the fact that there is a geographic distribution to multiple sclerosis, that the HLA genetic type is thought to predispose people through an altered T cell response, and that association with EBV (or speculatively some other environmental trigger) in their view all favor an autoimmune hypothesis for multiple sclerosis rather than a venous hypothesis (Khan et al. 2010).

They offer several points based on the known pathology of multiple sclerosis. They argue that while disturbed venous outflow could make it easier for immune system cells to migrate out into the brain tissue, thus causing inflammation, other acute or chronic brain diseases do not result in widespread demyelination. A further issue is that inflammation is not a feature of late MS, although older patients should have more significant stenosis and therefore more opportunity for immune system activity. Another important counterpoint in the view of the authors is that MS patients do not have occlusions of the retinal veins such as those seen in venous stasis retinopathy. Venous stasis retinopathy occurs when an artery in the eye crosses a vein and blocks it, causing damage in the area of the retina served by that vein. They argue that if the jugular veins were blocked, then patients should have the symptoms of venous stasis retinopathy. Instead, patients with MS have atrophy of the retinal nerve (Khan et al. 2010).

Other logic-based opinion includes the fact that increased cerebral venous pressure occurs in several other diseases, none of which cause multiple sclerosis. They also comment that transient global ischemia, mentioned earlier in this chapter, is a feature of jugular valve incompetence but not associated with MS. They further mention that in a variety of cancers or trauma, jugular veins are removed without people apparently developing multiple sclerosis. Finally, they declare that the cerebrospinal venous system is highly complex with multiple variations, collaterals and a lack of research clarifying the separation between the periventricular zone and the deep white matter venous flow. Given these facts, these MS researchers dispute the possibility that Dr. Zamboni could have identified abnormalities in all MS patients. Here is their opinion: "This raises further questions regarding the results of the study by Zamboni et al., who claim the ability to completely (100 percent) distinguish MS patients from controls with TCCS-ECD criteria established in their laboratory" (Khan et al. 2010).

These prominent MS researchers conclude that while Dr. Zamboni's work presents many opportunities to advance understanding of multiple sclerosis with a new direction for research, it must be considered very preliminary. They reiterate in their concluding remarks that duplex ultrasonography in the cerebrospinal system has no published consensus of standard criteria for normal venous return (Khan et al. 2010).

Many of the objections raised by these researchers were discussed earlier in this book. In other cases further research is needed to clarify how venous issues interact with the immune system in multiple sclerosis. The most prevalent theme through all published papers related to CCSVI, including Dr. Zamboni's, is that much more research is necessary before people truly understand how this pathology relates to the immune system activity and lesions in MS.

As was mentioned in chapter 1, scientific debate always includes this kind of back and forth. There will certainly be more papers on both sides of the argument as time goes on.

Plain-Language Summary and Comment

While Dr. Zamboni's "big idea" presented in the last chapter forms an interesting hypothesis, no one had ever thoroughly studied the blood flow in the venous system of the head and spine.

Dr. Zamboni's research team designed each study to build on the former study so they were able to develop their hypothesis systematically. The first study using their new technique showed only that people with MS have altered hemodynamics more often than controls do. The last study confirmed with venograms that the five-test protocol identifies changes in blood flow caused by physical venous malformations. The researchers tested 263 people with multiple sclerosis and 472 controls over the 3 initial studies, with only MS patients showing gross abnormalities.

A critically important follow-up study done by the Italian team of researchers shows that training is required to perform the five-test protocol successfully. Before widespread training is available people with MS seeking similar Doppler studies in local clinics in a desire to get ahead of the research may potentially pay for diagnostic findings that are essentially meaningless.

The five-test protocol is not widely accepted. People critical of Dr. Zamboni's work have questioned whether this diagnostic is valid and have focused on studies that seem to show it is not meaningful in addition to criticizing the unproven status of the technique. This is likely to be an area of hot debate in the medical literature for the coming years. The fact that Dr. Zamboni was able to discern MS patients from others suggests he has honed in on something unique in the blood flow of MS patients, but others need to learn to do this very problematic technique and similarly demonstrate this ability before skeptics accept it.

Another possibility that may establish the association of CCSVI with MS is Dr. Haacke's imaging protocol, which combines several types of assessments, including evaluating the brain with MRI, iron levels with SWI, the cerebrospinal blood flow with flow quantification and cerebrospinal system abnormalities with MRV. The data gathered will be pooled in a worldwide registry, and this information documenting large numbers of patients undergoing treatment may provide a breakthrough.

An important finding from SWI MRI research is that iron appears to be deposited backward along refluxing veins; this echoes Dr. Zamboni's comment on the importance of earlier research that showed the MS lesions expand in successive waves countercurrent to the normal blood flow. However, iron in the brain as identified by SWI is still an area of active research; neurologists have not accepted iron as a surrogate marker for multiple sclerosis.

The center of excellence concept, in which imaging centers all over the world participate in data collection using Dr. Haacke's imaging protocol, is a unique approach to gathering scientific evidence on a large number of patients in a short amount of time. It also provides an opportunity to refine the imaging protocol as data comes in so that findings and interpretation improve.

Replication has come from all over the world. In Dr. Simka's clinic, MS patients traveling to Poland for evaluation show CCSVI 90 percent of the time. A team in Jordan likewise confirmed CCSVI in 92 percent of MS patients but not in controls. In Kuwait, researchers who included both neurologists and interventional radiologists found CCSVI in 96 percent of MS patients while normal people revealed abnormalities only 7 percent of the time. This open-label confirmation from all over the world affirms the association of CCSVI with MS.

The early findings in from the large study at BNAC reveal CCSVI in the majority of MS patients even with technical difficulties in the phase 1 results. This study is ongoing and new cohorts are to be evaluated by updated and improved protocols over the coming months. The team at BNAC has already contributed immeasurably to the body of research related to CCSVI, with several studies on venous hemodynamics in relation to iron in the brain, atrophy, and cerebrospinal fluid flow all showing that poor blood flow is associated with these other problems.

MS is associated with CCSVI. There is enough evidence at this point in time that it is difficult to deny that this is a feature in many MS patients. The unanswered question is this: what does CCSVI have to do with the development of MS? Some speculate that CCSVI causes MS. Others believe that CCSVI triggers the MS autoimmune process. Others suggest it is merely an epiphenomenon and thus meaningless. It is a frustrating fact that more research is needed to answer these questions.

One way to find out if CCSVI plays a causative role in MS damage is for patients to have problems in their veins repaired and see if MS symptoms resolve to any degree. If patient MS symptoms improve over time, reflected in a reduced EDSS and/or MRI that show reduced lesion or iron loads, then this would suggest CCSVI pathology is related to MS damage itself and is not just a bystander problem of some sort. This kind of research is in the earliest stages, but there appears to be promise. Hopefully, Dr. Haacke's centers of excellence may contribute to the worldwide understanding of how treatment impacts iron loads, oxygenation and other objective parameters related to circulation in the brain as they work with the protocol and refine the approach.

There are many difficulties in moving from theoretical ideas to a reliable and successful treatment procedure that consistently works for patients. The next chapter will look at repair of CCSVI in the first patients who have been treated with the liberation procedure and variations performed by other practitioners.

6

Endovascular Treatment:
The "Liberation" Procedure

The right to life includes consenting to medical treatment—posted on TIMS

The research reviewed in earlier chapters, starting with the thread of historical evidence that MS has a venous component carried through to current-day work done by Dr. Zamboni, suggests that venous alterations are common in people with MS. The obvious possibility these facts raise is that venous blockages may play a role in the disease process that results in multiple sclerosis. In 2007, the Italian research team began the first study designed to evaluate how repair of malformed veins with an angioplasty procedure affects symptoms of multiple sclerosis. The research, reviewed in depth in this chapter, was published in 2009 (Zamboni et al. 2009b).

To review the pertinent terminology, angioplasty refers to inserting a catheter into the vascular system with the intention of repairing the blood vessel via that route. Technically angioplasty takes place in arteries and venoplasty in veins, though the more familiar angioplasty is commonly used for either. Patients have termed this the "liberation procedure" when used in relation to CCSVI.

Study of Angioplasty for CCSVI

The title of the study evaluating treatment of venous occlusions in people with MS is "A Prospective Open-Label Study of Endovascular Treatment of Chronic Cerebrospinal Venous Insufficiency" (Zamboni et al. 2009b). The Ethics Committee of the Ferrara University Hospital approved this study. *Open-label* means that no one was blinded in this study, which is typical for an initial study.

This study has caused considerable controversy, primarily because some patients interpret it as convincing in light of other research (such as that cited earlier in this book) that suggests MS has a venous component whereas critics have focused on the limitations of the study. Because of its importance, the following section describes this research in detail, with comments by the author of this book included to assist with the interpretation of technical information.

Patients and Procedure

Sixty-five patients with multiple sclerosis and evidence of CCSVI participated in Dr. Zamboni's treatment study. Thirty-five of the patients had RRMS, 20 patients had SPMS, and 10 patients had PPMS. These patients were treated with angioplasty starting in February 2007 (Zamboni et al. 2009c).

The goal of this study was to assess the safety of the angioplasty procedure as well as to evaluate how it affected some of the clinical features of multiple sclerosis. In order to see what influence this treatment had on MS, the researchers administered a series of tests before and after the procedure, as follows:

1. They evaluated cognitive and motor function.
2. They analyzed the rate of MS relapse.
3. They assessed the rate of MRI-active positive-enhanced gadolinium MS lesions.
4. They asked the patients to evaluate themselves with a standardized quality-of-life questionnaire.

Patients were evaluated about 18 months after the procedure. This study generated preliminary information regarding how treatment of CCSVI affects some MS symptoms.

Safety and Patterns of Stenosis

The Italian research team reports that, concerning the procedure itself, this group of patients did not have any unexpected complications. Angioplasty is a common procedure and considered relatively low risk (Simka et al. 2010c; MacDonald 2010).

The researchers noticed that there were combinations of stenoses across neck and spine major veins. They grouped these combinations as follows:

Pattern A: 30 percent of the patients had a pattern in which stenosis of the azygous was combined with stenosis in one of the internal jugular veins.

Pattern B: 38 percent had significant stenosis in both internal jugular veins and the azygous.

Pattern C: 14 percent had bilateral stenosis in the internal jugular veins and a normal azygous vein.

Pattern D: 18 percent had multilevel involvement of the azygous vein and the lumbar systems, and half of these patients also had an internal jugular vein that was stenosed. This pattern was seen in 9 of the 10 PPMS patients, but only 2 of 35 RRMS patients and 1 of 20 SPMS patients (Zamboni et al. 2009b).

Types of Occlusions and Morphology

The occlusions were of variable types. One item the researchers noticed was membranous obstructions of the veins. This means that a membrane of tissue that is not normally present had developed and was blocking blood flow.

The azygous vein was twisted in several patients. This research is the first to document twisted azygous veins in patients with MS. This malformation was relatively common in this group of subjects, with 12 of the 65 MS patients demonstrating this abnormality.

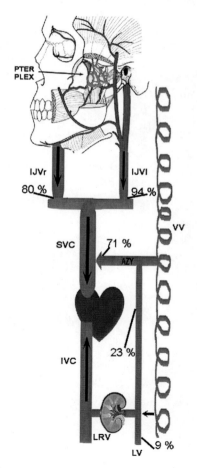

This schematic representation of the venous system is reprinted here with the permission of Dr. Zamboni. This was originally published in "A Prospective Open-Label Study of Endovascular Treatment of Chronic Cerebrospinal Venous Insufficiency" (Zamboni et al. 2009b). The curly figure represents the vertebral veins surrounding the spine, the heart shape represents the heart and the kidney shape the left kidney. IJV means internal jugular vein with either an L for left or an R for right. AZY means azygous, LRV left renal (kidney) vein, IVC inferior vena cava, and SVC superior vena cava. The pterygoid plexus is frequently the site of collateral circles. The percentages in this schematic represent the locations of the stenosis seen in the study (Zamboni et al. 2009b). This schematic shows the relationship of all the veins involved in CCSVI.

Stenosis in the internal jugular veins was usually observed as an annulus, which is to say a narrowing that goes all the way around the vein in a ring-like fashion. Another type of occlusion seen was a septum, a kind of dividing wall in the vein. The presence of a septum was frequently associated with valves that were not functioning correctly.

In some cases, these valves had actually developed upside down. Instead of the valve functioning to keep the blood from backing up into the brain (as with the Valsalva) the way it was supposed to, it was functioning to keep blood from escaping the brain.

The lumbar veins themselves were not usually malformed, but when they were, the most frequent problem was agenesia. Agenesia refers to the fact that the lumbar veins did not develop correctly or else they never developed. The lumbar veins are a long way from the brain, but when they are missing, the blood backs up through the vertebral plexus along the spine, burdening the vascular system all the way to the cerebrospinal system (Zamboni et al. 2009b).

This varied list of venous anomalies seen in the 65 patients brings to light one of the biggest issues challenging pioneering physicians working with this new model. Each of the venous problems listed poses a different technological issue for the person trying to detect and then repair the malformation, and each situation poses a different prognosis. In some cases, corrective repairs are not available — for instance, when the vein is missing (Zamboni et al. 2009c).

Pressures

As part of their study protocol Dr. Zamboni's team of researchers checked the central venous pressure in each subject by taking a pressure reading inside a large vein (the superior vena cava) near the heart (Zamboni et al. 2009b). This measurement established the baseline internal pressure for the person's overall venous system. However, the pressure of the entire *cerebrospinal* system in patients with CCSVI was slightly increased compared to their personal baseline. The researchers thought this was because all the veins in the cerebrospinal system freely communicate with one another in a complicated venous tree, and as some of the veins were blocked, the entire system was slightly burdened. The venous system is generally a low-pressure system, and other research has shown that differences of 2 to 3 cm H2O are significant and treatable, although such small differences would not be significant in the arterial system (Labropoulos et al. 2007).

When the Italian researchers checked the venous pressure on both sides of the stenosis, they confirmed that the pressure on the brain side of the stenosis was several points higher than the other side of the stenosis and also the

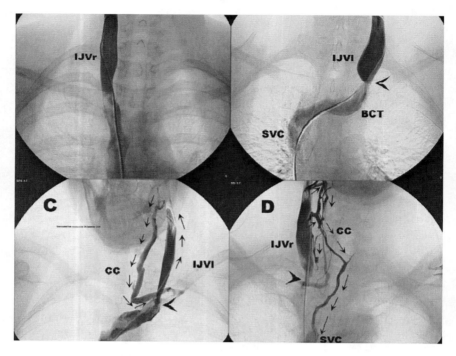

Venous abnormalities as seen with venogram. Image A shows a normal right internal jugular vein. Image B shows a left internal jugular vein with stenosis indicated with an arrow. Image C shows a closed stenosis of the left internal jugular vein with collateral circles indicated with small arrows. Image D shows the stenosis of the right internal jugular vein and activation of numerous collateral circles involving the thyroid veins; one of these carries the flow to the superior vena cava. Image originally published in "Chronic Cerebrospinal Venous Insufficiency in Patients with Multiple Sclerosis" (Zamboni et al. 2009c). Used with permission.

baseline measurement. Repairing the stenosis effectively returned the pressure in the system to baseline.

Repairs

Repairs were highly individualized depending on what corrections an individual person needed. The twisted azygous veins mentioned earlier were repaired with balloons in 11 patients; one patient required a stent to keep the twist open. All of the other stenoses affecting the azygous were repaired with balloon angioplasty. Ninety-six percent of these azygous repairs were still functioning well at 18 months, with the patients exhibiting free-flowing venous circulation.

Repairs in the internal jugular veins were not as reliable. Ninety-one percent of patients had a problem with the internal jugular veins, but the repair with balloon angioplasty did not last in 47 percent of these patients. This occurred usually about 8 to 9 months after the procedure. Dr. Zamboni mentions that stent insertion might prevent this restenosis. However, the fact that there are no stents designed specifically for use in these veins caused the team to err on the side of caution with the intention of repeating angioplasty procedures as needed.

The physicians were unable to repair agenesis of the lumbar veins, and people with this venous deformity were not able to have procedures to correct their cerebrospinal circulation. This meant that the 18 percent of subjects who were affected by this, most of whom had PPMS, continued to have impaired blood flow after treatment.

Results: How Treatment Impacted Multiple Sclerosis

Data for the 35 RRMS patients show some interesting statistics. Data among this group includes information about relapses. The results showed the following: 27 percent of patients with RRMS were free of relapse before their liberation treatment; 50 percent of these patients were free of relapse after their treatment.

The results also show that all relapses occurred in patients whose veins restenosed. No patient whose veins remained free of stenosis for the entire 18 months experienced a relapse. This important finding suggests there could be a connection between impaired blood flow and relapses.

Concerning MRI findings and gadolinium enhancement, the researchers found that 50 percent of RRMS patients had gadolinium-enhancing lesions before their treatment, and 12 percent had gadolinium-enhancing lesions after their treatment. Additional evaluations conducted on this subset of subjects showed that in comparison to evaluations done before treatment, there was a significant improvement in the functional composite score among RRMS patients following treatment. They also had improved scores on the quality-of-life questionnaire (Zamboni et al. 2009b).

Data for the PPMS and SPMS groups was less promising. In part, this may be because a portion of these people had venous issues that could not be addressed because of agenesis of the lumbar veins similar to that seen in the RRMS group. Additionally, this group of patients with progressive disease included individuals with jugular repairs that restenosed. The quality-of-life scores showed a significant improvement. However, concerning the functional composite score, there was an improvement at six months, but the difference compared to pre-treatment scores was not statistically significant at eighteen months (Zamboni et al. 2009b).

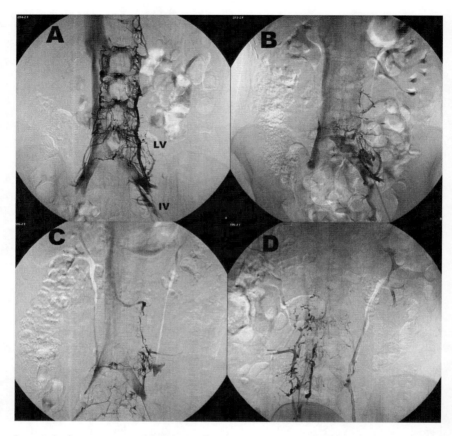

Image A shows a normal lumbar venous system with the hexagonal, ladder-like appearance when dye is injected in the iliac vein. The circulation is draining outward into the lumbar veins and upward to the azygous system. Images B, C, and D show a dramatic bare venous lumbar tree in MS cases with a combination of agenesia and atresia (veins never generated or else wasted away). This picture is further complicated by an associated stenosis in the azygous system and this combination of stenosis was associated with pattern D (the pattern that often accompanied progressive disease in their research). This image was originally published in "Chronic Cerebrospinal Venous Insufficiency in Patients with Multiple Sclerosis" (Zamboni et al. 2009c). Used with permission.

Summary

The team of researchers in Ferrara has given the world a new way of looking at multiple sclerosis. The initial treatment study is a promising start from which the rest of the research community can build toward results that are more conclusive. However, because it is an initial study, it has some limitations, as described in the next section.

Criticism of This Study

While many MS patients have embraced this study with hope, MS experts have focused on several weak points and urge a cautious interpretation. Dr. Zamboni himself says other researchers need to confirm this preliminary study and carry the research forward to more conclusive trials (AAN 2010).

CONCERNS ABOUT THE NUMBER OF RELAPSES • The visible disease course in multiple sclerosis fluctuates, with symptoms typically waxing and waning and periods of remission alternating with periods of relapse. Because of this, data regarding symptoms is extremely difficult to evaluate. One of the criticisms made against this study is that data compared people to themselves before and after the procedure, since there was no control group. In people with MS, inflammatory relapses decrease in frequency from year to year. Therefore, even ineffective therapies can appear to have some beneficial effect when evaluating only relapses before and after treatment (Murray 2005, 328).

CONCERNS ABOUT RESTENOSIS • Another problem mentioned by critics concerns the high rate of restenosis seen in treated subjects. If every vein that was treated remained free from restenosis, the results would have been clearer; if even a few people had relapses, it would be obvious that adequate circulation does not prevent relapses. Unfortunately, there were relapses and restenosis, so this required further analysis and interpretation of subgroup data sets.

Because the only patients who relapsed had restenosed, it suggests that restoring circulation to a free-flowing state may prevent relapses. However, there were only 35 RRMS patients. This is a small enough number that chance could have played a role, especially in MS, which is so variable.

CONCERNS ABOUT OTHER CONFOUNDING FACTORS • Any patient who was taking a disease-modifying drug before the study stayed on the drug during the liberation treatment study. Such drugs are widely considered helpful for reducing relapses and may have played an unknown role in the outcome of this study.

Another concern is that the placebo effect may have played a significant role since this study was open label; both the physicians and the patients were presumably hoping for a positive effect and this can influence the outcome in open-label studies (Turner et al. 1994).

Patients' Reactions

These kinds of concerns are expected following an open-label preliminary study; there is no way for a preliminary study to be conclusive. However, while the use of angioplasty to improve multiple sclerosis is a new concept, angioplasty to repair an occluded vein is an extremely common and relatively safe procedure (MacDonald 2010). Considering the long history of venous issues in multiple sclerosis — such as slower blood flow, demonstrated by reduced mean transit time (Adhya et al. 2006) — some MS patients interested in the CCSVI model felt this study confirmed the possibility that CCSVI influences MS. This was especially true of people for whom standard therapy was ineffective.

Some of these MS patients have decided that they would like to have their blood flow evaluated and any occlusions repaired via typical interventional radiology techniques. The logic they use is that good blood flow should be beneficial to the MS brain, no matter what causes it (Green 2010). While some critics have argued there is no evidence of CCSVI in multiple sclerosis patients (Sundstrom et al. 2010), other vascular physicians evaluating MS patients for CCSVI have identified impaired blood flow in the vast majority of patients assessed, as described in the last chapter. Many patients have already obtained treatment (see patient stories in the next chapter).

Presumably, some readers of this book are considering evaluation and potential treatment themselves. The next section discusses angioplasty, with special emphasis on facts that should be considered as part of that calculation based on patient reports following angioplasty procedures for CCSVI that have been done to date.

Angioplasty

Angioplasty has been around for more than 40 years and vascular specialists today consider it a routine procedure (MacDonald 2010; Yevzlin and Asif 2009). A review of the history of angioplasty offers a perspective on how this procedure evolved from a revolutionary idea to the most common medical procedure performed in the world today (Cohen 2004).

History of Angioplasty

The era of modern angioplasty began in 1964 when a physician named Charles Dotter, MD, began experimenting with opening narrowed arteries in legs by introducing progressively larger catheters into the narrowed area guided by a fluoroscope. Difficulty in reproducing the technique, complications in early patients, and resistance from some people in the medical community delayed acceptance in the United States (Cohen 2004). In the words of Martin Leon, MD, a leader in the field of interventional radiology:

The climate was hostile, antagonistic, disbelieving. I think that surgeons, internists, non-cardiologists felt that this was a very bizarre way to treat patients, that mechanical balloon barotrauma could not achieve durable results and could not achieve safe initial results. So skepticism would be an understatement of the overwhelming tide of sentiment in the early days [Leon 1998].

In 1967, Martin Judkins, MD, improved on the former techniques of angiography, which is visualizing the arteries using dye visible to a fluoroscope (the pictures created are called *angiograms* when performed in arteries). Dr. Judkins's innovation involved entering the arterial system through the large femoral artery in the groin rather than the arm, then advancing the catheter to the area to be evaluated. This is applicable to veins as well, with venograms using the femoral vein for access to the venous system. The Judkins technique is still used today (Angioplasty.org).

European physicians were quick to adopt and build upon Dr. Dotter's ideas. In 1974, a German physician working in Zurich, Andreas Gruentzig, MD, began developing the double-lumen (it has two channels) balloon catheter, which was an early version of today's balloon catheters used in angioplasty. He successfully created this catheter at his kitchen table. Dr. Gruentzig presented successful results with animal studies using his new balloon catheter at the American Heart Association in 1976 (Cohen 2003).

In 1977, Dr. Gruentzig presented the results of procedures with human subjects at the annual meeting of the American Heart Association. According to an informational website detailing the history of interventional radiology, this is what happened: "In September 1977, in Zurich Switzerland, Gruentzig performed the first coronary angioplasty on an awake human. Now, a year later, when he presented the results of his first four angioplasty cases to the 1977 AHA meeting, the audience burst into applause, acknowledging his breakthrough with a standing ovation" (Angioplasty.org).

This enthusiastic endorsement is understandable in the context of cardiac care at the time; coronary artery disease was a serious problem and technically very difficult to treat, requiring major surgery with all the associated risks. This innovation, which allowed treatment of a conscious patient in an hour or two and a surgical wound that was small enough to cover with a Band-Aid, was a fantastic leap in technology. Additionally, because this procedure was performed using an angiogram to guide the operator, the doctor knew immediately whether the procedure was successful (Cohen 2003).

Dr. Gruentzig carefully fostered the growth of the budding field of *interventional radiology* by establishing training and standards of practice, and fostering development of innovative devices to improve patient outcomes. He was able to establish a firm founding for the field before he tragically passed away in a plane crash in 1985.

From 1985 through 1993, companies catering to the new field invented and perfected many new devices for use in interventional radiology, including small tools that can remove tissue in an area rather than merely dilating the area with a balloon, catheters capable of measuring pressure in tiny vessels, intravascular ultrasound, and stents (a small device that holds the blood vessel open). Stents are an important innovation that improved the success of angioplasty because they reduced the rate of restenosis greatly. French physicians implanted the first stent in 1986 (Angioplasty.org).

In 1997, an important milestone was reached when over 1 million angioplasties were performed worldwide, making it the most common medical intervention in the world. By 2001, that number had increased to 2 million (Cohen 2003).

Interventional Radiology Today

Today's interventional radiologists (IR) receive formal training and must pass stringent board exams, as do members of any other medical specialty (Angioplasty.org). There are now areas of specialty within the field of interventional radiology as well.

Many different physical problems that used to be very dangerous and difficult to treat can be treated using interventional techniques today with virtually no trauma to the body or organs. Angioplasty has replaced a significant percentage of major heart procedures, has developed ways to remove a blood clot in the brain causing a stroke, can employ stents to prevent rupture of an aneurysm in the brain or the body, and can even intentionally occlude an artery leading to a tumor so that the tumor will die from lack of blood flow. This partial list should give the reader an idea of the scope of practice of the various specialties within interventional radiology. These procedures show how innovative IRs have found ways to use the vascular system as a kind of internal highway to correct a number of pathologies without having to dissect other healthy tissues to get to the operative site. Though this field is relatively young, it has become a cornerstone of modern medicine in the 35 years since the techniques first became available (Cohen 2003; Cohen 2004).

Patients Request Angioplasty for CCSVI

Patient interest in the angioplasty procedures for CCSVI created a huge demand for clinics with interventional radiologists or vascular doctors that could provide this type of evaluation and procedure.

Michael Dake, MD (Stanford)

As was mentioned in chapter 1, Michael Dake, MD, of Stanford University was asked to evaluate MS patient Jeff Beal for CCSVI. Dr. Dake was the first physician in the United States to undertake evaluation, then angioplasty, for CCSVI. What he discovered confirmed Dr. Zamboni's work in Ferrara, and he began an observational study of CCSVI by doing off-label intervention in other patients with MS when MRV confirmed stenosis. Forty patients were evaluated and treated in this observational study (Dr. Dake, personal communication, June 9, 2010; see also Dake 2010b). As of this writing, he is finalizing details on an IRB trial that will include a blinded control group (the people will not know if they got real treatment or sham treatment) (Dake 2010b).

Unfortunately, there were two complications among treated patients in the observational study — one stent migration and one patient on anticoagulation who had a stroke (discussed later in this chapter). These problems were described repeatedly in the press to characterize angioplasty for CCSVI as dangerous and to insist IRs should halt treatment (Samson 2010). As a result, researchers in a clinic in Poland undertook a study to evaluate the safety of interventional procedures in CCSVI, including stents (Simka et al. 2010c), discussed in the next section.

Marian Simka, MD, Euromedic (Poland)

Marian Simka, MD, of Euromedic, a private hospital in Poland, obtained approval from the Bioethical Committee of the Regional Silesian Board of Physicians in Katowice, Poland, and then began evaluating and treating patients for CCSVI at their request. Their medical team has maintained a commitment to contribute to the medical literature based on their experience.

Dr. Simka felt the initial pressing concern for the medical community was in regard to the safety of procedures undertaken to alleviate CCSVI. With this in mind, the clinic kept specific data regarding safety on a large number of patients treated in spring of 2010 so they could investigate the incidence of untoward events related to the procedures performed in their clinic.

PATIENTS TREATED • Their research paper is titled "Endovascular Treatment for Chronic Cerebrospinal Venous Insufficiency: Is the Procedure Safe?" and accepted for the journal *Phlebology* (in press). This paper details the treatment of 284 endovascular procedures performed on 276 people with multiple sclerosis and chronic cerebrospinal venous insufficiency. Dr. Simka and his team of doctors always use balloon angioplasty first and attempt to avoid using stents. In 159 cases, they used balloon angioplasty alone, but in 125 cases the patient required a stent (Simka et al. 2010c).

PATTERNS OF STENOSIS • The vascular areas that required repair in this study were slightly different from those detailed by the Zamboni team. This team saw occlusions in these areas:

39.4 percent of patients had occlusion of one internal jugular vein;
59.9 percent of patients had occlusions of both internal jugular veins;
6 percent of patients had occlusion of the azygous vein;
2.1 percent of patients had occlusion of the brachiocephalic vein.

In this series of procedures, there were no serious complications, and most notably, no stent migration. Dr. Simka deemed the procedures safe, as detailed in a letter to the Canadian Parliament:

> Recently in some neurological papers it has been claimed that surgical treatment for CCSVI can be dangerous. Interestingly, these statements were based only on the beliefs of the authors, and not on the body of evidence. Contrary to those opinions, in our clinic we have demonstrated that these procedures are safe and usually well-tolerated by the patients (sic) [Simka 2010c; see also Simka et al. 2010c].

Other Practitioners

Today, there are a growing number of other pioneering vascular physicians or IRs treating CCSVI all over the world. In some cases these physicians are doing off-label treatment (Grady 2010), in other cases they have undertaken observational studies, and in some cases individual governments have approved such treatments for their citizens (Al-Omari and Rousan 2010).

Interventional Radiology in CCSVI

Patients may wonder how IRs evaluate these occlusions, and how they know they are treating something of physiological significance. Some critics have suggested that the vascular physicians involved in this work are misinterpreting the hemodynamic situation in patients with MS when evaluating for CCSVI (Doepp et al. 2010). What follows is a review of how these evaluations are conducted.

Evaluating Stenosis

When a practitioner performs the angiogram or venogram and discovers a narrowing in the blood vessel, the venogram catheter also has the capability of checking the pressure inside the vessel. This allows the physician to evaluate the intravascular pressure on both sides of the stenosis to see what kind of an effect the occlusion has on the blood vessel. The doctor can also evaluate the area to see if the body has developed collateral blood vessels to carry blood flow around the blockage. This information, coupled with the image of the stenosis on the venogram and patient symptoms, provides direct evidence and supporting evidence that the occlusion is physiologically significant and should be repaired (Zamboni et al. 2009a; see also Labropoulos et al. 2007).

These evaluations can be repeated after the angioplasty or stent procedure before removing the catheter to make certain the intervention was effective. Pressure should return to normal and collateral circulation should disappear when the previously stenosed artery or vein is functioning normally. This gives the physician direct, immediate feedback about the procedure.

Interventions to Repair Occlusions

Dr. Simka evaluated the use of both balloons and stents in his safety trial. He also comments that in the future it may be clear that some problems may be better suited for open surgery rather than interventional radiology techniques (Dr. Simka, May 30, 2010, personal communication).

However, at this time, most CCSVI treatment is focused around the standard angioplasty techniques. These standard techniques include balloons and stents, as discussed in the following sections.

BALLOONS • There are a variety of balloons that the physician may use in angioplasty. The basic idea is that the physician advances the catheter to the narrowed artery or vein (visualized with the angiogram or venogram) and then inflates the balloon to stretch open the lumen of the vessel inside the narrowed area. The interventional radiologist has a variety of techniques to make this basic concept successful, from specialized balloons that can score thickened, stiff tissue so they can stretch more easily to balloons that can deploy a stent (Cohen 2003).

Angioplasty without stents widens the narrowed area without any permanent alteration in normal physiology and without long-term concerns. This is a very safe approach, and many IRs performing procedures in CCSVI choose to do simple balloon angioplasty for the safety of the patient.

The downside to simple balloon angioplasty is that stenosed areas may restenose after repair, sometimes very quickly, requiring repeat procedures. In some CCSVI cases patients were required to have as many as three or four repeat procedures (Grady 2010). In the search for a more permanent solution, industry innovators designed stents.

STENTS • A stent is essentially a flexible mesh tube made of metal that is very small and thin when collapsed. In its collapsed state, it is small enough to fit over the uninflated angioplasty balloon. The physician advances the balloon with the stent to the area of the narrowed blood vessel. He then inflates the balloon, which opens the stent. The stent remains in the open position due to properties of the metal. The balloon is deflated and withdrawn, leaving the stent behind. A second kind of stent is self-expanding and does not require a balloon to open.

The previously described study done by Marian Simka, MD, who has performed hundreds of treatments for CCSVI, documented safety data with regard to stent placement in the 44 percent of patients who required them (Simka et al. 2010c). He says he believes that over time perhaps 70 percent of patients treated for CCSVI will require stents, based on the percentage of patients with restenosis they are seeing in their clinic (Marian Simka, MD, May 30, 2010, personal communication). In his letter to Parliament Dr. Simka states, "In our opinion, precise preoperative diagnostics and selective use of the stents (if balloon angioplasty was not successful) can make the endovascular management of CCSVI free of significant complications and, in terms of restoring the proper venous outflow, more efficacious than performing balloon angioplasty in all cases" (Simka 2010c).

Dr. Simka states that, considering the young age of MS patients and concerns about long-term durability of stents (including issues of restenosis), they have maintained a cautious position regarding the use of stents and prefer to use simple balloon angioplasty where possible (Dr. Simka, personal communication, May 30, 2010).

Many companies manufacture stents, and stents can be made of different metals, but one metal that is frequently used is called Nitinol. A summary of the unique value of this material for stent applications in 2003 describes it this way:

> Nitinol (nickel-titanium) alloys exhibit a combination of properties which make these alloys particularly suited for self-expanding stents. This article explains the fundamental mechanism of shape memory and superelasticity, and how they relate to the characteristic performance of self-expanding stents. Nitinol stents are manufactured to a size slightly larger than the target vessel size and delivered constrained in a delivery system. After deployment, they position themselves against the vessel wall with a low, "chronic" outward force. They resist outside forces with a significantly higher radial resistive force. Despite the high nickel content of Nitinol, its corrosion resistance and biocompatibility is equal to that of other implant materials [Stoeckel et al. 2004].

This ability of Nitinol stents to return to the former memorized shape makes them especially useful in areas where there is a lot of movement, like elbows (Yevzlin and Asif 2009). This is at issue in CCSVI because some of the areas where the venous truncular malformations occur are in the neck, where movement is expected. Interventional radiologists may allow the patient to hold a stent when they are discussing angioplasty before the procedure. From personal observation, the stent is surprisingly soft and can be bent, crushed and twisted in any direction while still returning to the original shape and size. It seems impossibly resilient considering its extremely light and delicate appearance. Anyone considering angioplasty procedures that may include stents should ask for an opportunity to hold this device.

A newer innovation in the field of stent technology is drug-eluting stents. Although bare metal stents were designed to prevent restenosis, they may still restenose after they are implanted. This happens because as the lining of the blood vessel grows over the stent, the lining sometimes thickens, partially obstructing the blood vessel again. The drugs that coat the metal in a drug-eluting stent discourage this (Cohen 2010). A downside to drug-eluting stents is that they may require more anticoagulation than other stents, though researchers are still debating the ideal anticoagulation regimen (Cohen 2010).

Another downside to all stents is that they are permanent foreign bodies. Once the physician places them in the vein or artery and the lining of the blood vessel grows over them, they become part of the blood vessel. By the time a month or two has passed, the stent is fully incorporated and cannot be removed without sacrificing that section of the blood vessel. Because MS patients are typically younger than patients who traditionally might receive stents, the permanent nature of stents poses a particular concern. A stent will need to function for decades in an MS patient and since restenosis is relatively common in stents, there is good reason to be concerned.

The decision to agree to placement of the stent if the physician feels one is required should not be taken lightly. Patients must ask their doctor what he could do if their stent should restenose, how often they need to be monitored, what kind of long-term care is required (including anticoagulation), and what this might mean for them over the years. Once a stent has been placed, there is no going back, but innovation may change that.

DISSOLVING STENTS • An innovation that is set to revolutionize stent technology is the bioabsorbable stent offered by Abbott and already being evaluated in clinical trials. These stents are made of a drug-eluting poly-l-lactic-acid material that the body absorbs completely over a year or two. The name of the study (still in progress at this writing) is A Bioabsorbable Everolimus-Eluting Coronary Stent System for Patients with Single De-Novo Coronary Artery Lesions, which is shortened to the acronym ABSORB (Ormiston et al. 2008) for people interested in following the development of this idea.

This important innovation should eliminate the problem of having a permanent foreign body in the blood vessel. The stent was approved for limited use in Europe as of January 2011.

Anticoagulants (Blood Thinners)

When the lining of the blood vessel has been damaged, the body tries to repair it by forming a clot in the area. Angioplasty, particularly when stents are used, damages the lining of the blood vessel, so many physicians prescribe medication to keep the blood from clotting after the procedure.

These anticoagulants are commonly referred to as blood thinners, though they do not technically thin the blood but rather block factors in the blood needed for clotting, like platelets. These types of drugs prevent a blood clot from forming and occluding the artery or vein. They also prevent the formation of a smaller blood clot at the site of the angioplasty or stent that might then migrate to other areas of the body, causing serious complications like a pulmonary embolism.

Physicians have differing opinions about how much anticoagulation a patient needs after an angioplasty procedure. Factors such as the type of procedure performed, the individual patient's blood work, and which studies the physician finds most applicable influence the kind of anticoagulation that an individual practitioner may prescribe post-procedure (Cohen 2010).

If someone has simple angioplasty, they may only need a day or two of anticoagulation. If the patient has stents, anticoagulation may be required for a couple of months. Sometimes, the practitioner prescribes low-dose aspirin long-term following anticoagulation treatment. If a person has a drug-eluting stent, their physician may prescribe anticoagulants for as long as a year. Again, it depends on the practitioner and the situation.

Different anticoagulant drugs have different mechanisms of action to prevent clotting. While these drugs provide an important therapeutic benefit in preventing blood clots, the patient must follow the instructions provided with these medications to the letter to make certain their blood retains enough ability to clot to prevent problems with bleeding.

One common type of drug, warfarin, presents a special challenge to patients because of dietary restrictions. This kind of drug works by blocking the action of vitamin K. When taking a drug of this type, people must be very careful to maintain a diet with a stable amount of vitamin K; an increase in vitamin K–rich foods in the diet would make the drug less effective, possibly resulting in a clot. The reverse is also true; a decrease in vitamin K–rich foods could allow the drug to be too effective, possibly leading to hemorrhage. If a physician has prescribed this type of drug, the patient must take the dietary instructions provided very seriously; this is significantly different from other kinds of dietary instructions.

Medical management for people on anticoagulants can be very complicated, and this is why people need a physician in their community for follow-up care. With most medications, lab testing is necessary to make certain the physician prescribed the right amount of medication for the individual.

One more common lab test to monitor the ability of the blood to clot is the international normalized ratio (INR). This test identifies 1 as the length of time it takes a sample of blood from the average, healthy person to clot. If a sample tested on a patient takes half that length of time — in other words, it clots up very quickly — that person's INR would be quantified as .5, which would be reported as <1. People who are taking medication to prevent blood clots typically take the amount of medication that maintains their INR in the range of 2.0–3.0. If the INR result was too high, meaning the blood takes more than three times as long as a healthy person's to clot, the person would be at risk for spontaneous bleeding.

SAFETY WHILE ON ANTICOAGULANTS • Patients who are taking medication to prevent blood clots are at risk if they should be in an accident because it may be difficult to stop the bleeding unless physicians can counteract the drug. A medic alert bracelet alerts emergency personnel to anticoagulant medication in the event of an emergency.

However, accidents that are less dramatic also put people at risk. For example, a fall with a blow to the head or a broken bone while on anticoagulation therapy might result in excessive bleeding with potentially severe or possibly even life-threatening consequences. Preventing falls while on anticoagulation poses a particular challenge for people with altered mobility. They must take extra care to make certain they are safe, even if that means using the electric cart at the grocery store rather than using their cane as they usually might.

One patient on anticoagulation after stent placement for CCSVI died of a hemorrhagic stroke after going home (Samson 2010). Hemorrhagic strokes occur when there is an existing weakness in the vascular system of the brain and a blood vessel breaks. According to information reported in the article, this woman's mother had also had a hemorrhagic stroke (Samson 2010). This type of weakness in the blood vessel can be heritable but there is no way to predict vulnerability to such a problem or prevent it. Because she was on anticoagulation when she had her stroke, the stroke was worse than it would have been otherwise. The online community felt her loss deeply because she was an active presence and a staunch advocate for people with advanced disease, such as herself, having the opportunity to choose treatment.

Anticoagulation therapy is very serious. Patients must make certain that they are very clear about what is required of them to ensure their safety. The difference between angioplasty and stents includes different anticoagulation after the procedure. To become fully informed, patients should understand what kind of anticoagulation is going to be required post-procedure. Because different drugs work in different ways and have different requirements, patients must talk to their own physicians and pharmacists to get personalized support.

Other Interventions in Central Veins

In Budd-Chiari syndrome, the hepatic vein is impaired due to venous truncular malformations (as mentioned earlier). If untreated, this syndrome will destroy the liver because the occluded vein does not allow proper drainage. Device manufacturers have created stents specifically to be used in the hepatic vein for Budd-Chiari syndrome.

Similar to Budd-Chiari, CCSVI appears to be a type of venous truncular malformation (Lee et al. 2009) but one that occurs in the cerebrospinal system rather than the liver. Recent work in Dr. Simka's clinic on the venous occlusions his team had seen in MS patients also suggests that these are congenital occlusions (Simka et al. 2010b).

Many of Dr. Zamboni's patients have malformations causing occlusion in the jugular, brachiocephalic or azygous veins. Dr. Simka's documented experience confirms this clinical picture (Simka et al. 2010c). One may wonder if vascular physicians routinely repair these veins for other reasons, or if repairs in this part of the vascular system are revolutionary in some way.

In fact, IR physicians must repair jugular veins when they stenose following use of a central venous line. A central line is the name for an intravenous line placed for long-term therapy in a large vein of the chest or neck, usually jugular or brachiocephalic veins. Central lines are common in patients who need chemotherapy or dialysis. The constant use of the vein to administer caustic medication or dialysis often causes damage to the vein and induces the development of stenosis. In order for these very ill patients to continue lifesaving therapy, the IR must find a way to repair the vein.

According to a review of other studies evaluating the management of central lines used in angioplasty and/or stents done in 2009, "The role of stent placement in the treatment of central venous stenosis (CVS) is widely regarded as less controversial than in the peripheral veins. Indeed, the Society of Interventional Radiology (SIR) guidelines have indicated stent placement for central vein lesion. Some investigators have even argued that central venous lesions represent a primary indication for stent placement due to the poor outcome usually found with balloon dilation alone" (Yevzlin and Asif 2009).

Concerns Regarding Central Venous Procedures

Although IRs consider central vein stent placement routine, the IR has to use stents that were designed for use in arteries. There are no stents designed specifically for veins, with a shape created to prevent migration in venous applications. Additionally, MS patients need to live a long time with such stents, as opposed to the very ill patients who usually receive stents in central veins. These facts have caused Dr. Zamboni to take a very cautious approach and prefer simple angioplasty over stents for patients with MS and CCSVI.

The previously cited review mentions one study that documented two cases of stent migration when the vascular physician placed the stents in central veins (Yevzlin and Asif 2009). The researchers explain that veins ordinarily expand and contract with respiration, and this can allow stent migration. As mentioned, there has been one documented case of stent migration in treatment of CCSVI (Samson 2010).

Clearly, stent migration is possible when placing stents in central veins. One institution that reviewed data from five years of experience documents 27 cases of stent migration during that time. Twenty-six of the 27 cases were repaired with endovascular procedures, which is to say they retrieved the migrated stent with the same type of angioplasty balloon that deployed it. One patient during this five-year period had to have open-heart surgery to remove a stent that had gone into the heart (Slonim et al. 1999), as did the one person with stent migration documented in CCSVI treatment (Samson 2010).

CCSVI Treatment in MS: Positive or Negative

The demand for CCSVI treatment is a patient-driven movement. MS patient advocates have contributed a tremendous amount of anecdotal information about their treatment on Internet social networking sites and forums like TIMS. The vast majority of these anecdotal reports are positive, with many patients reporting profoundly reduced fatigue, improvement in bladder function, improved sleep (including fewer nocturnal trips to the bathroom), improved energy, a resumption of normal workloads and sometimes even a return to former levels of function. Occasionally, YouTube videos online have provided impressive visual documentation of what appears to be profound improvement in some individuals.

Naturally, critics have pointed out that placebo effects probably play a role in these positive outcomes (Levy and Lang 2010). However, others argue the degree of positive anecdotal evidence is far beyond placebo effects seen in other MS treatments and that it is disingenuous for critics to dismiss the large number of positive anecdotal stories by simply calling angioplasty treatment in CCSVI an especially strong placebo (Embry 2010b).

Yet angioplasty in CCSVI does not have universally positive results. Dr. Simka commented that he has seen patients who had relapses after an apparently successful procedure. This seemed to be particularly true if they were ill or stressed (Dr. Simka, personal communication). Another physician treating CCSVI, Dr. Siskin, commented in a presentation that he is seeing roughly 30 percent of treated patients with dramatic improvements, 30 percent with mild improvements and 30 percent with no apparent change in short-term follow-up (Symposium 2010). More research is needed to really understand the interaction between venous issues seen in multiple sclerosis and the immune activation in the MS lesion over longer time frames, as has been mentioned previously.

Reported Problems with CCSVI Treatment

The initial patients treated in a variety of settings did not have the benefit of experienced practitioners. Though experience in this area of medicine is increasing constantly, it will take time for CCSVI treatment to be consistent and for results to be predictable.

Patients posting in online forums have mentioned some problems with angioplasty treatment for CCSVI. What follows is a compilation of some issues these pioneering patients have reported.

Stent Migration

As mentioned earlier, a single stent migration in one observational study on CCSVI has been repeatedly mentioned in the media as a cautionary tale (Samson 2010; Grady 2010). The patient involved had to have open-heart surgery because the stent had traveled into the heart as it migrated with the blood circulation.

This stent migration may have occurred because jugulars function in concert with the vertebral veins in an unusual and positional way. When a person is lying down, the jugulars carry most of the blood flow. When a person is standing up, the vertebral veins carry most of the blood flow. The jugulars collapse and expand over a wide range of widths to accommodate this hemodynamic. This distensibility may have played a role in the stent migration.

In addition to the issue of migration, the unusual distensibility of the jugulars also poses a special challenge for assessment of the hemodynamics in this area. Many of the CCSVI practitioners presenting at a symposium in New York (Symposium 2010) mentioned that repairs in the lower jugulars often opened up what appeared to be stenosis in the high jugulars. These stenoses in the high jugulars often turn out to be areas that collapsed because of stenosis that had developed lower down in the veins, frequently a malfunctioning valve. Several physicians mentioned that they now look for this issue first.

Intimal Hyperplasia

Intimal hyperplasia is the technical term for the thickening of the blood vessel lining. This sometimes happens inside a stent and it may partially occlude the blood flow and require further intervention. Dr. Simka reports he is seeing this in some patients (Dr. Simka, personal communication, September 2, 2010). Complete occlusion of the stent may be unrepairable.

Spinal Accessory Nerve Damage

Another issue is that the jugular veins, the carotid artery, the spinal accessory nerve and the vagus nerve are all very close together. It has long been known that interventions in the neck, such as carotid endarterectomy (removing an occlusion in the carotid artery), can be the cause of iatrogenic spinal accessory nerve damage (Laska and Hannig 2001). Some patients receiving repairs of the high jugulars with stents also reported spinal accessory nerve damage that required physical therapy and rehabilitation.

The author of this book was one of these people. In my case, the spinal accessory nerve completely regenerated, though it continues to be something that requires rehabilitation to strengthen the involved muscles. Theoretically, even balloon angioplasty might cause this issue. An indication that the nerve has been damaged is extreme shoulder pain and weakness after the procedure.

Restenosis

Many patients posting their accounts online report restenosis and the need for repeat procedures. This seems to occur most often after simple angioplasty, but occasionally patients have reported restenosis in stents as well.

Thrombosis

One anecdotal report posted on the TIMS forum detailed that the person had experienced clotting of the entire jugular vein after a second balloon angioplasty. He/she speculated this was due to not receiving any medication to prevent blood clots. An emergency physician performed surgery to remove the blood clot in the jugular vein to prevent permanent occlusion.

Anticoagulation Problems

As was mentioned earlier, one person had a hemorrhagic stroke while on anticoagulation therapy after stent placement (Samson 2010). This is the death often mentioned as a cautionary tale in the media (Samson 2010; Grady 2010).

However, many patients reporting on the Internet have talked about difficulties keeping the anticoagulation regulated and monitored in the therapeutic range. Frequent trips to the laboratory, frequent adjustments of medication to keep the INR at the right level, and bruising with the slightest bump (which for many clumsy MS patients is common) left many people surprised at how complicated this element of their CCSVI treatment was.

Vein Problems

Dr. Zamboni documented that some people have agenesis of the lumbar veins. There is currently no available repair for this issue. A few other patients have also reported other factors, such as a missing or malformed jugular vein, that the physician could not repair.

Other Problems

As more people with MS are treated, unexpected issues may be uncovered. The list of problems covered in this book will not be comprehensive. Although angioplasty procedures are relatively safe, there are still chances for complications. The possibility of negative outcomes highlights the need for care in one's local community. Fortunately, it is getting far easier to find people who are able to provide CCSVI treatment.

Birth of a Specialty

Patient demand for treatment of CCSVI in multiple sclerosis has created a need for expertise in this field while it is still in development. Nonetheless, those practitioners who have begun observational studies and IRB trials or are practicing in countries where this treatment is allowed have begun to contribute to the medical literature so that physicians in other locales can understand what is being learned by these pioneers.

On July 26, 2010, physicians from all over the world who are performing these procedures convened in Brooklyn to share their findings with one another (Symposium 2010). This gathering of talent represented many of the people with experience treating CCSVI worldwide.

The day before this symposium, July 25, 2010, the International Society for Neurovascular Disease (ISNVD) formally elected its first Executive Committee. The Society was formed legally earlier in June by Dr. Haacke along with two other members, Dr. Zivadinov and Dr. Sclafani. Their next step was to create the Executive Committee for the first year, after which the members of the society would vote to fill any new positions. Dr. Zamboni assumed the role of the first president, Dr. Zivadinov the president-elect and Dr. Simka the vice-president. This is a tremendous advancement for patients with CCSVI because it offers a professional forum for all interested scientists and clinicians without any bias against the study of vascular problems in neurodegenerative diseases. It also means that experts in this field will be able to establish standards for patient diagnosis in areas such as imaging, practitioner training, and patient treatment. The first annual meeting is planned for the spring of 2011 in Italy (see www.isnvd.org for more information).

Out of respect for the tremendous patient activism and interest in CCSVI, founding physicians of ISNVD promised to set aside time at their annual meeting for an open question-and-answer conference that patients can attend (Dake 2010b). This physician-patient partnership may be a model for the future and is a concrete example of how the politics of medicine is shifting.

Transitional Phase: Evolving from New Model to Routine Care

Though angioplasty in this area of the body is relatively routine for other similar circulatory conditions (as mentioned earlier), and the Society for Interventional Radiology has released a position statement that supports CCSVI treatment in some cases (SIR 2010), comprehensive evaluations of research findings related to CCSVI in MS will take at minimum 5–10 years before this work is complete (Embry 2010b). This means that there is going to be an uncomfortable phase for some time during which patients who feel they are losing the MS battle may wish for assessment of CCSVI.

The following sections offer information that might be part of that calculation.

Developing Practitioner Skills

Finding a practitioner who has made a commitment to developing skill in treatment of CCSVI is important. Because interventional radiology is a field in which physicians are accustomed to adapting current techniques to new applications, many interventional radiologists with no knowledge of CCSVI may be willing to attempt evaluation and repair, assuming this procedure would be very straightforward. The experience of those physicians who have done the most work in this field has made it clear: assessment and treatment of CCSVI is anything but simple or straightforward, even though repair of similar issues is considered relatively routine.

In interview with CCSVI Alliance, Dr. Salvi, the Italian neurologist working with Dr. Zamboni, made this comment regarding incomplete treatment (English is his second language; quoted verbatim as documented by CCSVI Alliance):

> You have to study the lumbar plexus, the jugular veins, and the azygous veins. It is very important because I saw a lot of studies, only partial, so you can't say "liberation," or "full liberation." Only a few have liberated all the vessels, this is very, very important. And most of the failure are due to this [that is, to not understanding the entire venous system and not discovering/treating all of the stenosis] [Salvi 2010].

Because it is easy to miss these venous truncular malformations, this may result in incomplete and ineffective treatment for some patients even if the model is correct, especially when working with inexperienced practitioners. Dr. Dake has stated that he undertreated his first few patients (Dake 2010). Several presenting physicians at the symposium echoed this as well (Symposium 2010).

Differences in Technology

Similar to Dr. Zamboni, in Dr. Simka's clinic they have developed the habit of pinpointing areas for repair with duplex ultrasonography before surgery so they have an idea where to look for abnormalities that may appear invisible on the venogram, such as a flap of tissue that the catheter may push out of the way during the venogram. In their view, a combination of evaluating venous hemodynamics before the procedure with duplex ultrasonography and MRV, then venograms, offers the best chance of finding more difficult venous malformations (Dr. Simka, personal communication, May 30, 2010).

Other physicians have moved toward other technology and have begun to use intravascular ultrasound (IVUS) to evaluate suspicious areas of the vein from the inside (Symposium 2010; Dake 2010b). This tiny ultrasound device is introduced into the venous system with the venogram catheter. One MS patient who treated in Dr. Dake's observational study reported that he went in for a second procedure and Dr. Dake found a flap of tissue in the vein that he had missed in the first surgery. The IVUS uncovered this otherwise invisible anomaly during his second procedure.

Dr. Haacke is contributing to the database with his MRV protocol using SWI MRI, BOLD (blood oxygen level dependent MR), and flow quantification. The data generated by these technologies is objective and not prone to operator error. Using these techniques he has uncovered widely variant abnormalities in the venous system, including variants in types of reflux. In some cases, the entire vein refluxes; in other cases the blood is flowing down the vein on one side and up the vein on the other in a kind of circular reflux (Haacke 2010d). The precise clinical significance of these differences is not yet understood and still under investigation, but the hope is that these additional evaluations will improve the information available to the IR before doing a procedure.

Some practitioners preparing to evaluate patients for CCSVI are seeking training in Italy from Dr. Zamboni and Dr. Menegatti in how to properly do the five-test protocol. Patients may like to consider asking sonographers offering evaluation of CCSVI if they have this training given the documented need for such training to generate reliable results. Dr. Zamboni remains committed to the idea that duplex ultrasound is the best technology for evaluating CCSVI.

Differences in Practitioner Philosophies and Approaches

As was mentioned earlier, Dr. Zamboni checks for agenesis of the lumbar veins, assuming patients would want to know that this is a problem for them even though it is not repairable. He also examines the left renal vein, and checks for May-Thurner disease; in his view, problems in these other areas burden the venous system and complicate CCSVI. However, not all practitioners check for problems in these other areas.

Another thing that has become clear is that there is a huge difference in ability to detect problems in the azygous vein. Dr. Zamboni's study, cited earlier in this chapter, states 86 percent of patients had azygous issues (Zamboni et al. 2009c). Dr. Simka's safety study states 6 percent of patients had azygous issues (Simka et al. 2010c). Dr. Dake likewise confirmed that he had identified azygous problems roughly 6 percent of the time in his observational study on 40 people (Dr. Dake, June 9, 2010, personal communication).

Dr. Haacke is refining his protocol for evaluating the azygous vein with

MRV. As of this writing, his team is improving their ability to detect abnormalities in the azygous with MRV by comparing venograms to the MRV interpretation that was made pre-procedure (Haacke 2010d). The hope is that data from this evaluation prior to an IR beginning angioplasty will improve patient outcomes. This ability to detect azygous issues via MRV is evolving but may end up providing the needed understanding about this vein and its role in CCSVI.

The physicians who specialize in this treatment will eventually establish practices that will improve the consistency of patient care. Patient outcomes will get better as physicians in this field clarify how they should evaluate these more difficult areas.

These issues highlight the nature of today's CCSVI evaluation and treatment. Because of this, many people, including Dr. Zamboni, have asked patients to look for IRB-approved trials.

Dr. Zivadinov has likewise encouraged people to seek treatment only in IRB-approved trials (Laino 2010). Many other neurologists have also insisted patients must be involved only in IRB-approved trials (Stanbrook and Hebert 2010; Samson 2010). Considering it is expected to take some years to fully understand how these venous issues contribute to MS, some patients may wonder how to find such a trial locally. Fortunately, this is going to be far easier than people imagine.

Institutional Review Board Trials

While it is true that the day will come when treatment is widely available and practitioners have experience, until that time participating in a trial is the best approach for people seeking evaluation of CCSVI. At first blush, the insistence that MS patients seek IRB trials seems impossible. For example, Dr. Zivadinov's treatment study had 8,000 people waiting and 30 spaces available when it began (CTV 2010a).

In addition to Dr. Zivadinov's study, the Vascular Group in Albany, New York, is enrolling patients for their approved trial. As of this writing, there are also several other trials pending approval in scattered local communities (see chapter 8). Patients interested in participating in a trial locally can check the FDA's website (http://clinicaltrials.gov) for current listings.

However, both E. Mark Haacke, PhD (Wayne State University), and David Hubbard, MD (San Diego, Hubbard Foundation), have applied for nationwide IRB approval. Dr. Hubbard's IRB was unconditionally approved September 2, 2010 (see chapter 8). Dr. Haacke is collaborating with Dr. Hubbard and providing the imaging protocol for their IRB.

This means that interventional radiologists in other communities can join this nationwide IRB-approved trial and their work will be part of that trial. The local interventional radiologist has no need to obtain his own IRB approval. If a patient with multiple sclerosis has an interventional radiologist that they have been speaking with in their own community, they might like to ask that IR to join this trial (see chapter 8).

Reasons to Be Involved in a Trial

In the future treatment of CCSVI may be routine. Until that time, participating in an IRB trial makes certain that the patient's needs and rights are respected. While angioplasty is a well-understood technique, its application for venous stenosis in multiple sclerosis is an off-label use and the influence such treatment may have on MS itself is unknown, even if it demonstrably improves circulation. This means information about how improving blood flow influences MS symptoms over time is critically important for the medical community.

Trials are often conducted for the benefit of a third party — for example, a pharmaceutical company or possibly a physician who wishes to publish a paper (Dr. Hubbard, personal communication, September 10, 2010). People choose to participate in trials presumably because they believe the new approach will help them. The institutional review board makes certain that the disclosures and documentation provided to the patients who participate in such a trial are very clear and there are no false claims about possible benefits.

Documentation provided to the patient in an IRB trial also makes the risks very clear. This helps the patient make decisions but it also protects the physician doing the procedure from any claims later that the patient did not understand what they were signing up for. This provides an important benefit in that practitioners who may have been reluctant to consider evaluating people for CCSVI could suddenly find themselves very interested in participating in this groundbreaking work.

Another important reason to participate in an IRB trial is that the information collected from every medical case contributes to the medical literature. This makes participation in such a trial an important contribution to the evidence base.

As mentioned, there are several IRB-approved trials currently recruiting patients. However, because the nationwide IRB-approved trial allows widespread enrollment of interventional radiologists in local communities and it is expected to be ongoing, the next section discusses this trial specifically.

Participating in a Trial
with the Haacke Imaging Protocol

The Hubbard Foundation IRB-approved trial, which can be made available in local communities nationwide, uses the Haacke imaging protocol. This approach applies comprehensive evaluation using MRI technology to assess how treatment impacts oxygen levels and blood flow in the brain. Patients are evaluated before and after angioplasty treatment, then again at 6 and 12 months, to assess changes in blood flow and oxygenation. Dr. Haacke will enter the data in a national registry providing a huge database that will hopefully prove the value of liberation-style treatment concerning blood flow, assuming the IR who performed the angioplasty procedure was able to provide complete repair of stenosis. MRI scans done under Dr. Hubbard's IRB trial will be sent to Dr. Haacke, who will then evaluate the results objectively.

Dr. Haacke makes this comment regarding the value of this protocol for patients undergoing a procedure for CCSVI:

> Having an MR scan prior to treatment is crucial for a number of reasons. First, it gives you a baseline of the brain tissue, MS lesions, vascular anatomy, flow characteristics, small veins in the brain, possibly perfusion in the brain if that is eventually added to the protocol, iron content, and the presence of any microbleeds or thrombus. Apart from the critical issue of acting as a treatment planning guide for the interventional radiologist or vascular surgeon, this information is the baseline from which you can judge what happens in the future. Do lesions go away, does blood flow improve, does iron content stay the same or reduce after treatment? Further, if complications develop, then this baseline scan can help determine where the problem lies. All this is not possible if you do not have the initial scan run with both the conventional imaging and the CCSVI protocol [Dr. Haacke, personal communication, September 12, 2010].

Note that the Hubbard foundation IRB does not mandate any particular angioplasty protocol for the interventional radiologist performing the treatment for this trial. Angioplasty is an FDA-approved technique, but this is an off-label use. The IR doing the angioplasty procedure will evaluate the cerebrospinal system and provide intervention on a case-by-case basis according to his or her best judgment and experience regarding repair of venous malformations in this area of the body.

Hopefully the Haacke imaging protocol will generate objective data that demonstrates angioplasty for venous malformations manifesting as CCSVI improves blood flow. From the standpoint of basic physiology, good blood flow, tissue perfusion and oxygenation should benefit the MS brain regardless of the cause of MS, providing it can be achieved.

Another way to have blood flow evaluated before and after angioplasty treatment would be to participate in the BNAC Self-Referral Program. This program includes Zamboni-style Dopplers to evaluate blood flow as well as MRV to look at the anatomy of the veins (see chapter 8 for contact information). This program is also keeping a database.

The existence of trials provides a way to get evaluation and treatment of blood flow issues related to CCSVI before it is widely accepted as a contributing factor to MS. But some people have looked to medical tourism in an effort to simply get the work done, presumably imagining that a simple trip overseas will solve their problems. The next section discusses this briefly.

Medical Tourism

Unfortunately, the lack of easy access to angioplasty for CCSVI has created a boom in pay-for-service entrepreneurial medical clinics. *Medical tourism* is the phrase that has been coined for patients traveling overseas to get treatments that are not available in their home country. Patients receive angioplasty for an out-of-pocket fee in these clinics.

Dr. Torrence Andrews sums up the problems with medical tourism while providing a logical argument for off-label treatment in local communities right now ahead of scientific certainty about the CCSVI/MS model.

> What we find is that while we are trying to do research that patients are going elsewhere to be treated ... I am not denigrating those programs [overseas clinics providing liberation-style treatment] they may be extremely good programs for all we know but there are problems inherent with medical tourism; you don't know who your doctor and your health care team are going to be, you don't know what their qualifications are, you don't know whether the equipment they're using is the state-of-the-art, the costs can be high and hard to predict, and what happens if there's a complication? What happens if during your procedure something goes wrong and you need prolonged hospitalization and you find yourself a continent away from home and family and you are in a very difficult situation? And then where do you go for follow-up if you've gone to Egypt to have your venous angioplasty procedure done and you have questions or complications or you think you have a recurrence; are you really going to go all the way back to Egypt [sic]? [Andrews 2010].

Dr. Andrews's quote really covers all the bases. Some people reporting their overseas CCSVI treatment experience on the Internet have said that they had a very positive experience. Yet some others have had problems and difficulty trying to resolve these issues far from home. Patients very commonly report needing repeat procedures. Receiving care in one's own community is safer and provides a means for ongoing care.

Plain-Language Summary and Comment

While there is ample anecdotal evidence on the Internet discussing benefits of angioplasty for CCSVI, this chapter offers a frank discussion of concerns and issues the MS patient interested in CCSVI should keep in mind before seeking evaluation and treatment from a vascular physician.

Patients who receive treatment today will get the best treatment the practitioner can provide within the constructs of these parameters:

1. The quality of the imaging and diagnostics done before angioplasty to guide the practitioner to areas of venous obstructions;
2. The practitioner's experience in evaluating and treating CCSVI;
3. The practitioner's understanding of what other pioneers in this field have learned to date;
4. The practitioner's willingness to assess for and discover malformations that may not be obvious;
5. The devices and tools available to the practitioner and their skill in using them;
6. The patient's individual presentation and unique physiology.

Clearly there are many ways to have incomplete treatment. This poses a dilemma for many patients interested in the CCSVI model.

On one hand, assuming CCSVI plays a significant role in or even causes MS lesions, treatment at the earliest possible opportunity would be desirable. On the other hand, patients with early MS can afford to wait until physicians know how CCSVI influences MS and how to evaluate and reliably treat these issues. Potentially, a person with very early MS, by waiting a mere year or two, may be able to take advantage of innovations such as dissolvable stents, which could provide benefits for the rest of their lives.

People in this situation might consider watchful waiting. During the time of watchful waiting, patients could engage their health with an eye toward the possibility that venous issues play a role in the disease. A few safe and simple measures might be considered with the advice of your physician:

1. Eat a heart-healthy, low-fat diet with many fruits and vegetables. This type of diet has a long track record proving its value in maintaining vascular health.
2. Consider consulting your physician about the possibility that supplements such as fish oil and antioxidants may aid in the effort to support vascular and endothelial health.
3. Exercise and avoid stressful situations, especially those that cause tight, shallow breathing; the thoracic pump, which is engaged with deep breathing, aids return through the venous system.

The decision to change watchful waiting to actively seeking consultation with a physician regarding treatment can always be revisited if the situation changes.

However, there is another group of patients. These people have been living with MS for long enough that they have developed progressive disease and have exhausted all standard treatment options. For such people the risk-versus-benefit calculation may be very different.

Such people should have a frank discussion with their own healthcare provider about how participation in a trial would affect their personal situation, including the possibility of needing anticoagulation post-procedure and how that would be managed given personal limitations.

Is it reasonable to imagine going to the lab once or twice a week, every week, for several months? Can falls be safely avoided for the period when anticoagulants would be taken? Perhaps avoiding anticoagulation is needed, thus dictating balloon angioplasty alone with only a few days of anticoagulants? These factors must be evaluated with individual healthcare providers for a personalized plan of care suited to individual needs and situations.

In addition, it's important to consider that treatment for CCSVI is still in the early stages of development. Is it understood that it's possible for treatment to be incomplete in spite of the IR's best effort? Will participation in a trial impose an onerous burden financially, considering patients will have out-of-pocket expenses? What if repeat procedures are necessary? Some people may want to wait, considering these limitations.

It must also be said: people must protect their hearts. Recall that the hallmark of progressive disease is loss of nerve tissue. While improved blood flow might maximize the possibility for healing, it would be unrealistic for people with progressive disease to expect function to return to pre–MS levels.

A neurologist from Dr. Zamboni's team, Dr. Salvi, stated, "I never saw patient in a wheelchair get up and walk away after the procedure, and this is very important for people to know. But in many patients the quality of life was better, and in many patients some improvement in body function was present. So there are few patient[s] who won't benefit in some [way] from CCSVI treatment [even if that just means to slow or halt progression], though this is just my opinion. The bedridden patient, I think, or I hope, that this can help with this patient [sic]" (Salvi 2010).

This hopeful comment suggests perhaps angioplasty for CCSVI may change progressive MS from a situation of constant nerve loss to one that is stabilized. These things will be studied over the coming years. In the interview cited above, Dr. Salvi continues by saying that patients treated in their first trial, the 65 patients of their open-label treatment (begun in 2007), continue to do well (Salvi 2010).

The author of this book has secondary progressive disease. I typed this book with one functional hand, with the aid of dragon-speak software, and while rotating my position from lying in bed so my feet wouldn't swell too badly to sitting in a chair on a Roho cushion to prevent my body from becoming too sore. When I talk about progressive disease, I am also referring to my personal situation. Yet even I feel cautious hope; not progressing would be a success in my view. The story of my CCSVI treatment is described in the next chapter, along with those of other individuals with MS. These encouraging anecdotal stories give MS patients reason to hope that angioplasty for CCSVI will become a routine part of MS care in the future and that these procedures will make a huge difference in patient outcomes.

7

Patient Stories

Carpe diem — posted on TIMS

Chapter 1, in the section titled "What Happened on the Internet," described how the patient forum on TIMS was the birthplace of what has now become a worldwide movement to demand immediate and thorough investigation of the CCSVI model. Within a short time, in response to patient demands, the MS Society urged that funds for research along this line become a priority in 2010 (see chapter 1).

Early discussions on the TIMS forum emphasized learning about venous insufficiency — that is, the ways that diagnostic tools could confirm this finding. In addition, discussions focused on how the evidence supporting venous insufficiency might be associated with disease development and progression in multiple sclerosis. Scrutiny as well as skepticism ran deep. In the spirit of critique, online posters intently discussed and dissected Dr. Zamboni's research reports and also evaluated the papers prepared by other scholars that he referenced to support his argument. After the initial skepticism accompanying most new views, many members of the forum felt his argument had merit and went on to seek evaluation and treatment. In fact, many of the early posters on the TIMS board eventually became involved in Dr. Dake's observational study, as mentioned previously.

Members of the TIMS board are rightfully early pioneers because of their involvement in this work. These patients have offered to share their anecdotal experiences with CCSVI in this chapter in a more comprehensive fashion than the reports they've posted on the TIMS boards. Most of the stories included here relate the experience of people treated more than 18 months ago. Anecdotal reports were not cherry-picked to represent successful outcomes. The following anecdotes were included because they give the most balanced view of current CCSVI treatment outcomes.

Stories from Stanford

Dr. Dake began observational study of CCSVI in patients with MS in May 2009. He was the first person in the United States to undertake evaluation of patients with MS for an associated problem of CCSVI. When he discovered diagnostic evidence supporting the finding of CCSVI, he repaired the responsible stenosis in accordance with the principle that good blood flow is necessary for the health of the associated organ.

Particular symptoms that many MS patients experience (general malaise, cognitive problems, fatigue, headaches, "stuffiness," heat intolerance) are similar to those experienced by people with acute jugular thrombosis or superior vena cava syndrome. Patients with these conditions have venous occlusions in neck and chest veins, and such occlusions require treatment that subsequently relieves these symptoms (Dake 2010a).

Dr. Dake was very clear in his discussion with the author during preoperative evaluation appointments. Other patients reported similar accounts and recalled that Dr. Dake emphasized that he could offer no guarantee that treatment would affect the course of MS. He stressed that too little research was available to make any conclusions about the association, including whether normal people might have similar venous malformations and occlusions. Nonetheless, he stood by his offer to treat based on the value of good circulation and the possibility some symptoms may be alleviated by the delivery of adequate oxygen to the affected areas.

Patients posting on the TIMS board knew that the whole concept of CCSVI and its treatment was a new idea. However, those patients who opted for CCSVI interventional treatment wanted the best blood flow possible for their MS brains regardless of how the research would eventually come out.

Jeff

Jeff, who was introduced in chapter 1, was the first person treated by Dr. Dake at Stanford in his initial observational study. Here is the rest of his story.

Jeff was diagnosed with relapsing remitting MS in 2007. Although he was diagnosed fairly recently, for 10 years prior to that time he had suffered from depression, sleep apnea and fatigue. His first relapse left him with bladder problems and intermittent severe headaches. At diagnosis, his MRI showed 21 distinct lesions. Although he still remained very functional, with an EDSS estimated at 1.5, he experienced leg pain and spasms that bothered him on a daily basis, in addition to the other symptoms. Soon after his MS diagnosis, he started taking glatiramer acetate at his neurologist's urging and he was still being treated with this drug when he opted to have treatment for CCSVI. In May 2009 Jeff underwent his first evaluation for CCSVI and subsequently was treated for this abnormality by Dr. Dake.

The MRV revealed bilateral jugular occlusion high in Jeff's neck at the level of the jaw with extensive collateral circulation that indicated a significant stenosis. Dr. Dake inserted two stents in Jeff's jugular veins, one on the left and one on the right. Although Jeff experienced moderate nausea and headache following the procedure, these symptoms resolved within a couple of days. In addition, Jeff experienced a slight accessory nerve issue causing moderate shoulder pain, which resolved over nine weeks.

When he went back for his two-month follow-up, imaging tests revealed that the tissue at the end of one of the stents had thickened and was partly occluding the blood flow. Dr. Dake repaired this occlusion with a simple angioplasty procedure. Jeff did not experience any of the symptoms or issues that had accompanied his initial stent procedure.

Following Jeff's initial stent procedure, his wife Joan immediately noticed that she had her "old husband back." Jeff was no longer so exhausted that he was unable to engage in evening social activities. In fact, he actually suggested they have a party at their house, something they hadn't done in a couple of years. In the months following his procedures, they went to baseball games, and Jeff was able to resume some of his former activities; for example, at their weekend home Jeff was able to chop wood in 90° heat. This is something that would have been completely impossible prior to his surgery. His headaches improved, his heat intolerance vanished, and his fatigue had completely dissipated. However, one thing had changed for the worse; Jeff developed a faint tinnitus, a whooshing sound in his ear that caused this award-winning musician problems, and the headaches, while milder, began occurring daily.

Dr. Dake evaluated the situation in November 2009 and discovered that the emergence of tinnitus was related to the blood flow in the jugular. Jeff and Dr. Dake discussed the problem and decided that the situation should be evaluated with a venogram. As a result, Dr. Dake performed another angioplasty and also noted that Jeff has a narrowing above the stent in the transverse sinus, which unfortunately he was unable to repair.

In spite of this anomaly Jeff continues to do very well 18 months after the procedure. He has had no exacerbations and no new symptoms related to his MS. His MRI reveals no new lesions. He very rarely has leg pain. He continues to have excellent energy levels and no longer experiences the profound fatigue that used to hamper his life. More than one year after his original stent procedure, he is able to vigorously exercise daily and has happily been able to maintain his preferred weight with his activity level. He sleeps deeply without the frequent nightly bathroom trips he used to endure and wakes up refreshed and feeling awake. His headaches are far less frequent than before he was treated for CCSVI and more manageable.

Jeff's angioplasty has made a positive difference in his life. Seeing Jeff's changes firsthand has motivated Joan to continue to advocate for increasing the availability of angioplasty for CCSVI by being active in CCSVI Alliance and moderating a Facebook page about CCSVI (http://www.facebook.com/pages/CCSVI-in-Multiple-Sclerosis/110796282297?v=wall). As Joan frequently tells others, the medical community needs to learn more about the role of CCSVI in MS and how to treat it. It's through the efforts of people like Joan that CCSVI and the liberation procedure are gaining recognition among patients and physicians alike. The MS patient community is indebted to her efforts.

Marie

As the author of this book, I've hinted at my own experiences with CCSVI treatment for MS in earlier chapters. Here I'll relate my story in greater detail.

As the discussion of CCSVI on TIMS evolved toward seeking evaluation, I contacted my local university, the University of Washington, and convinced the head of the vascular surgery department to evaluate me for CCSVI. During the examination, he saw evidence of venous reflux suggesting I may have the newly described condition. However, he did not offer any treatment solutions or suggestions for this problem.

After Jeff's treatment, Joan told Dr. Dake about my situation and he said that he was interested in evaluating my reflux as well. My husband and I were delighted to have this opportunity. After more than 15 years of living with MS, and being then out of options, I was interested in exploring the possibility that I may have CCSVI and hopeful that treatment might help me.

I was first diagnosed with RRMS in 1993 after a strange episode of tingling and stiffness from the waist down accompanied by a feeling of being off balance. Two years before my MS diagnosis, in 1991, I had been diagnosed with rheumatoid arthritis. Consequently, at the time of my MS diagnosis, I had already taken a variety of drugs intended to suppress my immune system, like methotrexate and plaquenil. When glatiramer acetate was introduced for MS, I went on it immediately. This drug controlled my inflammation very well and happily it relieved the joint pain I experienced with rheumatoid arthritis as well.

My neurologist repeatedly said I was a glatiramer acetate success story. Yearly MRIs revealed a stable lesion load and no evidence of inflammation.

However, that wasn't the whole story; I was still jogging at the track several times every week when I started on the drug in 1997, but by 2003 I was using a cane and couldn't jog to save my life. By 2008, my new neurologist diagnosed SPMS and I was using a rollator, a walker-type device, around the house.

As an RN and as a patient searching for answers, I had been collecting medical literature related to the idea that MS was degenerative and not primarily autoimmune for some time; this personal library of medical literature that I collected over the years was the resource for the early chapters of this book. It was very clear to me that managing inflammation, while somewhat effective in reducing certain symptoms, was not the same as managing MS. Consequently, I found Dr. Zamboni's theory that MS might be related to venous insufficiency compelling, and I was delighted that Dr. Dake would evaluate me for CCSVI as he had Jeff.

My initial evaluation with Dr. Dake showed that my MRV was very similar to Jeff's; I, too, had high jugular stenosis. My jugular veins, which should be about half an inch in diameter, were pinched to the size of linguine noodles at the level of my jaw. I underwent angioplasty with bilateral high jugular stents in May 2009.

Due to the years I suffered from MS without effective treatment, I'm considered a very disabled person. Because of this, I did not expect to experience a great deal of change after my procedure. In earlier chapters I explained how nerve loss in progressive forms of MS is permanent. Although I was willing to believe that over time some nerves might potentially regenerate (especially if CCSVI causes MS damage), my more realistic hope in terms of treatment outcome was for my MS disease progression to stop.

What did I experience? In fact, as expected, my impaired walking did not change after the procedure. However, I experienced many other important changes that really changed my quality of life. About two months after my procedure I realized that I was no longer plagued by flexor spasms. Consequently, I was able to stop all antispasmodic medication and even slept without spasms at night.

Prior to my procedure, flexor spasms had ruined my chance to use a nerve-stimulating device that improves drop foot (the inability to lift the foot). My flexor spasms had been so severe that my trial with the device failed. After the procedure, I was able to successfully use the nerve stimulator and I purchased one.

The profound improvement in sleep that I experienced was similarly dramatic. Instead of getting up to go to the bathroom every hour, then being unable to fall back asleep, I found myself sleeping deeply. I slept soundly enough to dream and sometimes I even slept all the way through the night uninterrupted. I felt refreshed and awake during the day, and my primary care physician commented that I looked 10 years younger; the drawn grayish pallor I had become accustomed to vanished. This makes sense anatomically because the facial vein is drained by the jugulars and mine had been blocked before the procedure.

These positive changes were very important to me. Having progressive MS, after my procedure I experienced my first positive outcomes in a very long time and the psychological as well as physical effects were beneficial. However, it's important to acknowledge that, along with the positive effects, I developed a few complications.

The first complication was rectus sheath hematoma. This was basically a very large bruise in the muscle of my lower belly where doctors inserted a catheter into the femoral vein. This was very painful and took many weeks to resolve completely. I was on bed rest for much of this time because it was so painful to stand up.

Another problem that I had was with spinal accessory nerve damage. When the stent opened, the nerve got pinched. An electromyogram (EMG) revealed that the nerve was regrowing and it would take roughly 9 months to a year for it to completely regenerate. It did regenerate, but during the time when it was damaged I had a lot of neck and shoulder pain. I believe that this may always be a risk for people who have interventions in the very high jugular area because of the proximity of the accessory nerve.

And finally, I had a lot of problems with anticoagulation and ended up getting lab tests twice weekly. Because of the accessory nerve issue I was uncomfortable driving for about 4 months, so this required someone else to take me to the lab for appointments during the two months I needed them. I also had many bruises on my body related to the anticoagulant therapy because I tend to plunge into the walls as I walk down hallways or lean into the door jambs as I pass through. It was rather dramatic and I looked like someone who had been in an accident of some kind. I also felt fatigued while I was on anticoagulation. Fortunately, this phase of therapy only lasted for two months. Dr. Dake recommends that his patients continue to use baby aspirin daily, and I still do this.

At my one-year follow-up, the MRV revealed that both stents are doing fine. However, my left jugular vein is stenosed both above and below the stent. I only have blood flow on one side, and there appear to be some abnormalities in the transverse sinus. I will soon be traveling to a facility that is doing the Haacke protocol to evaluate my blood flow with the flow quantification diagnostic technique.

I am a living example of incomplete treatment. I am anxious for the day when this condition is well understood and easily evaluated, and treatment is clear. Follow my story on Facebook or CCSVIbook.com.

Sharon

Sharon was the third person treated in the observational study at Stanford. Sharon's first event of MS probably occurred 35 years ago when she had a sudden feeling of being off-balance and tinnitus, but she was not diagnosed with MS until 2003. Her MS is secondary progressive, and her EDSS before surgery was a 4.5. Sharon never took any of the standard medications because her type of MS is not helped by standard therapies; she had no inflammation and no gadolinium enhancement on MRI. Since all of the standard pharmaceuticals for MS suppress immune function to stop inflammation, this would not be considered helpful for her. Consequently Sharon had no treatment options. She did use low-dose naltrexone (LDN) in the hopes it could prevent or slow disease progression.

Sharon loves to golf and attends Pilates classes several times every week. She started using a nerve stimulator in 2008 and found that it helped with her drop foot so much that she put it on every morning and only took it off at bedtime. She even took a trip to China using this device. Unfortunately, even with the stimulator, by 2009 it was becoming difficult for her to walk and she was beginning to trip again.

Sharon was happy when she was allowed to travel to Stanford and participate in Dr. Dake's observational trial. At 67 and retired from her position as CFO of a manufacturing company, Sharon felt that if she could slow or stop progression she could continue to enjoy her active lifestyle. Because there were no other available standard therapies for her, she felt she had nothing to lose; she decided before she even arrived in California that she would opt for treatment if she had any occlusions in her veins and treatment was offered.

When Dr. Dake did an MRV of Sharon's neck he discovered that her left jugular was over 99 percent occluded for a distance of 3 inches. He initially put in one stent to open this occluded area, but the blood flow didn't return until he inserted a stent in a damaged valve lower in the vein.

Following her CCSVI therapy, Sharon didn't have any dramatic changes initially. However, over time subtle things began to shift for her. Her nerve stimulator seemed to be working better, with effects comparable to those she experienced when she first began using it. Sharon's improvement was so significant that on many days she didn't even put it on in the house. Then one day she was at the chiropractor and he commented on the fact that she was there without the device! She was surprised to realize she left the house without it. A year after the procedure she continues to be able to take short errands out of the house without the formerly constant aid of the nerve stimulator.

At her one-year follow-up, the blood flow had decreased in the left jugular in comparison to how it flowed immediately after her first procedure. She is currently scheduled for a second venogram.

Sharon's story has a significant twist, however. She has two grown daughters, and not long before her angioplasty, one of them asked her if she got an electric feeling and sharp pain in her neck when she tipped her head. Suspecting her daughter was perhaps experiencing something similar to Lhermitte's as the first symptom of MS, Sharon was very concerned. She asked Dr. Dake if he would be interested in evaluating both of her daughters to see what could be learned. He agreed.

Carrie

Though both of Sharon's daughters were evaluated, only one of them turned out to have a venous occlusion in the cerebrospinal system. It was Carrie, the daughter who had experienced the electric feeling, who eventually was diagnosed with CCSVI. Other symptoms she experienced that could be attributed to MS or CCSVI were tingling hands and unusual fatigue. When she had a standard MRI of her brain, the radiologist discovered that she had several lesions in her brain typical of MS even though she had not been diagnosed with multiple sclerosis.

Carrie and her husband decided she should undergo treatment. In her situation, one jugular vein was crushed against one of her vertebral bones. This area was stented, and though she had spinal accessory nerve damage initially, today she is doing well. She chose not to consult with a neurologist and has not been formally diagnosed with MS.

Mark

Mark's MS story began in 2004 when he experienced severe optic neuritis and extreme fatigue. After several relapses, he got the official MS diagnosis in 2008. His radiologist numbered the lesions in his brain as "less than 15," although he did have a very large enhancing lesion in the frontal lobe. Mark's other symptoms included heat fatigue, depression, loss of balance, and dizziness. He also experienced problems with his thinking: he had a complete inability to concentrate, a loss of short-term memory and inability to maintain a conversation, and disorientation in busy places like malls. Mark's neurologist prescribed an interferon drug when he was diagnosed.

This 40-year-old father of young children estimated his EDSS at 2, and he had experienced something between two and four exacerbations. He felt that his MS progression was picking up speed, and his speech was slurred.

Mark's diagnostics before his CCSVI procedure revealed significant stenoses in both jugulars. The left and right jugulars were occluded at the ear level, with the left also occluded at the clavicle level. As part of his CCSVI therapy, he had 3 stents placed in the left vein, and one up high on the right. Immediately after the procedure, Mark experienced the kind of shoulder and neck symptoms that other people had reported, though by eight weeks post-procedure these were completely gone. As a result of this therapy Mark was one of those lucky people who experienced a profound change. His fatigue was almost completely gone, and, as he puts it, his "mental acuity is STEL-LAR, short-term memory improved 100 percent, no more balancing issues, no more wall rubbing, no stumbling, no tripping, no running into things." He also says that his depression has lifted and he feels that his outlook is now bright. He did, however, experience increased tinnitus in the right ear after his procedure, which was diagnosed by an ENT as venous hum.

Nine months after his original procedure, Mark went back to Stanford to have this tinnitus further evaluated to see if it was related to the altered blood flow. Dr. Dake did a venogram with the assistance of an intravascular ultrasound. He discovered a flap inside Mark's right jugular vein at the clavicle/valve level that was completely invisible to the venogram and MRV. This flap was vibrating with the pulse and was very long. High above this area, there was a stenosed area with the pressure gradient of 4mm/Hg. When Dr. Dake repaired the flap, the upper area opened up and the pressure gradient disappeared, along with the collateral network. Consequently, Mark's tinnitus was immediately reduced to near-imperceptible levels.

Mark makes a comment that gets to the heart of the issue for treatment of CCSVI: "Final thought, everyone is different in their MS and guaranteed you will be different in all ways when it comes to Funky Vein Syndrome, after 4 stents we thought this was licked except for the upper stenosis, but lo and behold, a bugger of a malformed valve can cause a pressure gradient to appear up high, collaterals and the like, despite the fact that another nearby stenosis had been stented already [sic]."

Today, Mark feels well, and his neurologist is very excited about the progress he sees in Mark's condition. There have been no new lesions on MRI, and no losses in his visual-evoked potentials. Importantly, he is able to do things that before were impossible. For example, he hiked up a steep hill solo in the summer heat with a group of kindergartners at a school picnic, carrying his three-year-old and holding the hand of another child. This was quite a feat for a person who previously had trouble thinking in noisy or confusing situations.

Mark has a video online of his venogram. It shows how repair of the vein caused the collaterals to disappear. This can be accessed at http://www.you tube.com/watch?v=cwc6QlLVtko.

Melissa (Mel)

Mel had an aggressive case of multiple sclerosis. Though symptoms appeared to come on suddenly, Mel had been having mild misattributed MS symptoms for years. These included depression (originally diagnosed in her teenage years), severe bouts of constipation, heat intolerance, and balance issues. What ultimately brought Mel to medical attention was a sudden case of double vision. An ophthalmologist and neurologist who initially evaluated Mel confidently reassured her that this was likely of no consequence, since she, a geneticist working at a renowned medical school and someone who ran 3–5 days a week, was too healthy to have anything significant.

Mel's first MRI, at 31 years of age, revealed that she already had two black holes among her eight lesions. One of these lesions was on her brain stem. Mel's neurologist placed her on interferon immediately. Unfortunately, she suffered from many of the side effects common to the interferon and the medication did not appear to be having a positive effect on her MS. Within 6 months of being diagnosed, Mel had more than five severe relapses, each of which left her bedridden for several days, and these took their physical toll. She had left-sided weakness, extreme fatigue, heat intolerance, clonus (a kind of spasm), worsening constipation, occasional incontinence, lack of balance, and emotional instability. Because her multiple sclerosis was so aggressive her treatments were likewise more aggressive than most. Unwilling to accept the advice of her then-neurologist, who suggested waiting until a better treatment became publicly available, she and her fiancé, Jamie, traveled to Johns Hopkins in 2008 to be evaluated for high-dose cyclophosphamide, a type of stem cell transplant that is still under investigation as a treatment for MS.

Cyclophosphamide is a type of chemotherapy that wipes out the immune system when given in high doses. As with most ASCT, this is a chemotherapy that usually makes people lose their hair and recipients must be hospitalized in protective isolation to make sure they are safe; for a period of time they have no functional immune system. After all of the immune system cells have been gone for several days, the patient receives stem cells harvested from their own blood before the chemotherapy. This rebuilds a new, naïve immune system. This approach is based on the autoimmune model of MS described earlier in the book.

After undergoing this experimental treatment, Mel felt some improvement. Her fatigue eased and she wasn't as intolerant of heat. Unfortunately, after several months it was clear that old problems were returning. They consulted her physician at Johns Hopkins and even though her MRI revealed she had no inflammatory activity in her brain, it was clear to him that she was progressing.

Mel decided that, rather than undergo her second chemotherapy, she would seek evaluation from Dr. Dake. Now 33 years of age, she was interested in the new theory. Her EDSS was 1.5.

Mel's MRV revealed that she had three jugular veins. On the left side two of them twisted around each other. She also had a congenital malformation in her transverse sinus; it was very small. In addition to this, her dominant right jugular vein had a stenosis. She had developed extensive collateral circulation as her body tried to compensate for the inadequate venous drainage. Dr. Dake placed stents in the high jugular area on both sides and the collateral circulation disappeared. He was unable to do anything with the transverse sinus and he considered it too risky to try.

After her procedure Mel had neck pain for about a week and then recovered completely. The most wonderful thing was that, in her case, response to the therapy was immediate and profound. The fatigue dissipated, her emotions stabilized and she no longer needed any antidepressants. She began running on the treadmill again, and before long was taking time for a run *after* work! For someone who used to have such profound fatigue that getting through the day was a challenge, this was a dramatic change in lifestyle.

Mel continued to do well until late May and early June 2010, when the unbearable heat of Houston summers returned. Mel noticed increasing fatigue, some balance issues, and a constant pins-and-needles feeling in her left hand. Mel was already scheduled for her annual follow-up with Dr. Dake in July 2010. At this visit, MRI/MRV revealed some narrowing of the left jugular vein, below the stent on that side. Dr. Dake was hopeful, though unsure, that opening up that part of the vein could alleviate symptoms. Mel underwent an angioplasty on the left jugular vein on July 9, 2010. All MS symptoms disappeared within days of the procedure. At the time of this writing, the only detectable remnant of MS is that her eyes don't track properly when tested, though she had to get a new prescription for her eyeglasses; the old prescription was too strong.

For MS patients, perhaps the most amazing comment from Mel is that she now feels normal.

Following the chemo, I felt well, but still always felt like I had MS. After the stent procedure, I felt like I did before MS changed my life. I felt normal for the first time in years! Though the decisions Jamie and I have made can be seen as somewhat unconventional, it is what was right for us at the time. I feel that I have attacked my MS from all angles: the chemotherapy helped address the autoimmune components of MS while the CCSVI has addressed the vascular component. Remember that you are your best advocate. Always fight for the treatment you feel is best for you, even if it may go against standard medical advice.

Sammyjo (Sam)

Sam's onset of multiple sclerosis was violent and dramatic. Diagnosed in 1995, this CEO of an online financial services company had to take steroids for her relapses several times a year. She went on glatiramer acetate the year it came out, and to her great relief only experienced one more relapse.

Unfortunately, her MS continued to progress, and by 2002, she was diagnosed with secondary progressive multiple sclerosis. Her neurologist recommended mitoxantrone. After seven doses of this drug, Sam's heart function showed a 10 percent decrease, and her neurologist stopped the medication. Sam experienced no relief in her MS from the drug. Too disabled to continue working, she moved across the country to be near her family. She felt like she was dying. Her new neurologist placed her on an interferon drug and monthly steroids. Yet this approach was not helping either; she needed a new approach to dealing with her disease.

That's when Sam got what she calls her first "get out of jail free card": low-dose naltrexone, or LDN. She had a motorized wheelchair on order when she started this alternative therapy, but soon found she didn't need it. In fact, she was able to walk without a cane.

This respite lasted until 2007, when her ability to walk began to deteriorate again and she had to go back to a cane. By this time, both of her legs were severely weak. By 2009, when CCSVI sprang onto the online MS patient community, she was ready to think in a new direction.

Sam traveled to see Dr. Dake and he discovered that she had bilateral stenosis in the jugular veins as well as a problem with the valve at the bottom of the jugular where it twisted around the carotid artery. She also had extensive collateral circulation. She had three stents placed bilaterally, and her collateral circulation disappeared.

Sam was one of the people who experienced spinal accessory nerve damage. In her case, it took seven months for her neck to feel comfortable again. She had extensive physical therapy during that time. Another problem she experienced was a menses that lasted 17 days while she was on anticoagulants. She became so anemic that she ended up in the emergency room. She stopped taking the anticoagulants at that point.

Despite the side effects, Sam felt improvements immediately. She was able to walk up and down a 30-foot hall in her home without a cane and found that her energy rebounded to old levels; she began visiting friends and attending events outside her home again. Another important improvement in her quality of life is that for the first time in many years, she found her constipation had cleared up and she was regular. Within two months nighttime myclonic leg spasms and the painful morning extensor spasms stopped.

Sam went back for a follow-up 10 months after her original procedure. There were some changes in her blood flow, and she was noticing increasing extensor spasms. Her team of doctors decided that she should have another venogram. Dr. Dake, using his growing experience, discovered several areas of stenosis not treated in the first procedure, including some in the azygous area. The stenoses were not severe but needed treatment with three more angioplasties.

Other practitioners have commented that their opinion of what should be treated has evolved over time: several of the physicians presenting at the symposium in Brooklyn stated that they undertreated patients initially and are seeing better results now (Symposium 2010).

Sam had no negative side effects from her second procedure, and it was performed on an outpatient basis with only a 4-hour recovery time. She is feeling improvement in symptoms again, and is very glad that she got to participate in the early discovery phase of CCSVI treatment.

Sam has more information about her treatment online at http://www. healingpowernow.com.

Lew

Lew is a manufacturing engineer whose hobby was competitive racquetball prior to his diagnosis. Something of a fitness nut, Lew put a lot of stock in his physical abilities. He also enjoyed maintaining his very large yard in a park-like state. Diagnosed in 2001, his MS was fairly progressive, and by 2005 he was diagnosed with SPMS.

Lew had started out with an interferon, but continued to have relapses and disease progression. He participated in the Tovaxin (Opexa) trial, and discovered he was one of the lucky participants that got the real drug after the first year was unblinded. He was in the trial for a year and a half; however, this revolutionary approach did not help his condition and, surprisingly, he feels he worsened at a more rapid pace after entering the trial. His neurologist then prescribed natalizumab. Unfortunately, he continued to progress while on that drug as well. By 2009, he was using a cane and his physician assigned his EDSS at 4.5.

Lew had to be very careful to avoid becoming overheated, and care of the beautiful yard was becoming extremely difficult; as soon as he got warm, his vision got blurry, so others took over the task of lawn care. His bladder had stopped functioning properly and he also had to catheterize himself at bedtime.

When Lew had his MRV at Stanford, it revealed a double jugular on one side. It also showed stenosis in both high jugular areas. Each area was stented as part of his CCSVI therapy. A week after this procedure was completed, Dr. Dake contacted Lew at home and said that when he returned for his follow-up he would like Lew to consider a second repair; after thinking about Lew's double jugular and studying the venograms and MRV, Dr. Dake realized that repair was possible. Lew agreed to have this second repair. While it may sound like it would work well, the "double jugular" needed repair because it carried very little blood flow. This turned out to be due to a non-functioning valve in one of the jugulars, and an inverted valve in the other. Dr. Dake placed a stent in the middle of the inverted valve and the return of blood flow through the area was immediate.

Like some other patients with stents in the high jugular area, Lew developed spinal accessory nerve damage from his original procedure. This resolved over the following 12 months. He experienced no problems at all with his second procedure.

However, he did experience improvements that were evident right away. Lew no longer needs a cane. He is working full time and puts in an average of 50–60 hours per week, with a good deal of it on his feet. He reports that he is completely wiped out at the end of his long days but he also recovers far more quickly than he did before his procedure. These days, he even has enough energy for evening activities.

His only complaint is that since he has secondary progressive MS, there is neurodegeneration and many long-held symptoms are still with him, even though they are not progressing at this time. Lew hopes that some other regenerative strategy will help restore some of that lost function. Lew says, "The word 'cure' is not in the vocabulary of this stent-o-neer until a repair mechanism is found and I can go back to exercising strenuously and not having to void my bladder so often [sic]."

Around the time of his one-year follow-up appointment Lew began to think perhaps his heat sensitivity was returning. He took this feedback to Dr. Dake and a new MRV image revealed terrific blood flow through the stents, but Dr. Dake noticed something that was unusual: Lew's brachiocephalic vein was stretched around his trachea, causing a slight narrowing. However, after sharing these images with other IRs who are treating CCSVI, it was decided not to intervene at this time.

Lew considers his procedure a great success. He can mow the huge lawn without severe consequences if he does it in three "chunks," whereas prior to his procedure he was unable to mow the lawn at all. Another example that demonstrates the changes Lew has experienced is that he went through the airports on his trip for the initial procedure with a cane and had to be in a wheelchair most of the time. During the visit just before the second procedure he only used his cane. Ninety days after the second check-up he didn't even bring his cane. He has now actually *lost* his cane. He says that for the first time in the nine years since his diagnosis, he can say that the last six months were better than the previous six. Here is a section from his blog post in September 2010:

> I created this blog about 14 months ago to track my progress through the CCSVI procedure, sometimes called the liberation procedure. It has become completely evident that the "rush" of things to be on high alert for after the procedure, things like improved heat intolerance, improved walking, etc., has been relegated to simply monitoring myself for myself's sake. The shine is off the procedure, I've been given my gold star at my one year check up, and my jugulars are flowing freely as they are held wide open by stents. So what happens from here is not only going to be very gradual, but also simply the consequence of me living my life. In other words, the treatment/procedure I had done is not "active" anymore like it was at the beginning when I was really noticing some profound improvements. I mean I put my cane away, how huge is that? I still don't need it by the way.

Follow Lew's blog posts at http://myhopefuljourneyintoactualmsrecovery.blog spot.

Summary

These stories reflect the best big-picture view of treatment as it stands right now. Providers are still working out details, such as whether a double jugular needs to be treated, or whether an abnormality at the brachiocephalic is acceptable, and whether problems in the transverse sinus can or should be repaired.

Note in Mark's story that when a flap missed in his first surgery was later repaired, an area high in his jugular suddenly functioned correctly. These are the kinds of things that can only be learned as practitioners work with people. This kind of thing cannot be learned on animals and cannot be studied in the laboratory.

It is important to understand that all of the practitioners in this field are learning from one another and practitioners gain experience as they treat more patients. Please keep in mind when evaluating this model that even the most experienced practitioners do not have expertise or any possibility of guaranteeing success even if the model is correct.

These particular stories were also selected because of the wide variety of treatments these individuals used before they elected to participate in the observational study of CCSVI. No one can say that these patients didn't give standard therapy a fair shot. The fact is that the standard drugs were failing these patients and they were losing the battle. They elected to participate in this early work because in their personal situation a new approach was their only option.

A Story from Italy

Gianfranco Campalani

Gianfranco Campalani is a cardiac surgeon practicing in Belfast who was diagnosed with PPMS in 1986. Originally from Ferrara, Italy, he went back to visit and his brother arranged a meeting with Dr. Zamboni in July 2006.

Dr. Campalani was fascinated by Dr. Zamboni's novel approach to MS. His specialty as a cardiac surgeon gave him an advantage in understanding the vascular system. The theory made sense to him, and he was delighted to have an opportunity to undergo Dr. Zamboni's highly specialized duplex ultrasound examination the next day.

Dr. Zamboni identified several blockages in Dr. Campalani's veins. In August 2006 Dr. Campalani had the liberation procedure performed, watching the procedure with a vascular surgeon's eyes and marveling at the findings.

Before the procedure, Gianfranco could walk with a cane no more than 50 yards. His weaker leg was difficult to lift and he struggled. But he says that within five hours of recovering from his procedure he was able to walk in the hall without his cane, which caused his partner to cry with joy. He felt stronger, walked taller, could lift his weak leg better and his bladder function improved. He continued to work in Belfast as a cardiac surgeon, even being featured on television as one of Northern Ireland's "Superdocs."

In 2009, however, he began to notice some of the symptoms creeping back. The old weakness was starting to return. He asked his colleague to do a venogram and they compared the results to images from his original liberation procedure. Sure enough, the same veins had restenosed. The stenosed areas were treated once again and Dr. Campalani had the same positive response to treatment that he had the first time.

Recently Dr. Campalani saw Dr. Zamboni and they learned that while the right lower jugular remained free flowing, the left lower jugular had again restenosed. Dr. Zamboni's fellow researcher and interventional radiologist, Dr. Galleotti, treated the left lower jugular. This was the third angioplasty Dr. Campalani had in 4 years on that area.

Dr. Campalani's diligence in seeking evaluation has paid off; he says that he continues to feel strong and is free of progression four years after the original procedure. This is an amazing feat for someone with primary progressive MS

24 years after initial diagnosis. He continues to work as a cardiac surgeon in Belfast.

Dr. Campalani is now an outspoken advocate for patients being allowed treatment using this relatively safe approach. He said in an interview:

> I believe that when a new treatment has practically only minor possible complications (as reported by Zamboni with venogram and angioplasty) and a good potential for benefits, as opposed to the pharmacological treatment rich in harmful side-effects, the need for rigorous scientific double-blind trials is nonsense. We need a few more intelligent and courageous vascular surgeons and radiologists to start treating vascular anomalies (strictures of the jugular veins) on their own merit, not mentioning MS. But the medical establishment is notorious for being conservative and generally lazy [O'Shea 2010].

Summary

Dr. Campalani's story was included for two specific reasons. Dr. Campalani is a cardiac surgeon and has a superior background for evaluating the liberation procedure. His willingness to undergo the procedure and endorsement of the approach speaks volumes.

The second reason is to emphasize that ongoing evaluation is important and repeat procedures may be necessary. However, this story also offers great hope for the progressive patients because Dr. Campalani's four years of stable MS is very surprising considering his diagnosis. It's difficult to argue that this might be some kind of "placebo effect."

Stories from the Hubbard Foundation IRB Trial

Because patients have the chance to join in David Hubbard's nationwide IRB-approved trial by asking a local IR to participate, the following stories of two people treated using this approach are included, though they were necessarily treated recently. Devin is Dr. Hubbard's son.

The imaging protocol used in this trial provides the interventional radiologist objective data about how the angioplasty procedure influenced blood flow. This information allows the operator to evaluate whether they accomplished complete treatment.

Devin

Devin is the owner of a marketing research firm. Because he uses a functional MRI in the course of his work, he leases time on the machine from his father's foundation and works in close proximity with his family. Unfortunately, starting in 2006 this got very difficult because Devin felt inexplicably frustrated and irritated all the time. He would lash out irrationally, causing everyone stress and pain. He suddenly had no sense of humor and was constantly angry. It became such a problem that the whole family was in counseling to try and understand what dynamic caused such a change in his behavior.

Devin also had been experiencing something that he calls "locked up." By that he means that when he was in busy or confusing situations, he became incapable of making a decision, even if it concerned something completely inconsequential. He would become so stressed he would turn and leave with no explanation.

However, it turned out to be more than a psychological issue. In May 2009, Devin, 26, woke up to discover that one half of his face was paralyzed. He was also experiencing double vision. Devin went to the hospital, where the neurologist diagnosed acute disseminated encephalomyelitis (ADEM, discussed earlier in this book). This self-limited disease clears up on its own and usually leaves no remaining deficit.

Devin, however, wasn't so sure. He was told if he had a second incident, he would then have the diagnosis of multiple sclerosis. The second incident came in December 2009.

He had an MS hug, severe Lhermitte's, another round of double vision, and severe pain in his skin; even a T-shirt hurt. Devin's parents both sought to learn everything they could about MS to help their son.

For his part, Dr. Hubbard, a neurologist himself, was surprised to discover that MS was still a disease of unknown origin. He was disappointed so little progress had been made in the field in spite of the fact that pharmaceuticals were now available.

Devin's mother, Arlene, came across CCSVI in the online MS patient community. Dr. Hubbard realized they could use BOLD technology to evaluate Devin's blood flow in his brain. Devin's blood flow was clearly abnormal, and as a result Dr. Hubbard became committed to investigating the new model thoroughly.

A local interventional radiologist treated Devin. He discovered that Devin's azygous was severely occluded, as was one internal jugular vein. These were repaired with angioplasty.

The next day Devin knew something was very different. He felt lighter — he smiled and laughed. He felt calm, in control, and able to think clearly. He was completely changed.

Four months after his procedure, he continues to do well. He says he is the calmest person in his family now. All of his MS symptoms are gone except a very mild double vision when he looks to the extreme of his peripheral vision. The Lhermitte's is gone. He can exercise as hard as he likes without triggering any symptoms and even has the balance to stand on one foot and tie his other shoe.

Devin has become an advocate for other people to have the opportunity to be treated. He feels like he has himself back.

Danielle

Danielle is no stranger to venous malformation; she was born in 1976 with a red area on the bottom of her foot that was misdiagnosed as a cavernous hemangioma (a superficial vascular lesion usually found on the faces of infants and very young children that usually resolves with time). When she reached puberty, this anomaly suddenly began growing. Danielle describes it as being similar to a cluster of grapes under her skin on the bottom of her foot. This made her foot extremely painful to walk on. At 11, the physician evaluating the situation identified as it a venous malformation and suggested that the best way to manage it might be a partial amputation of her foot. She and her parents decided not to do this, and she lived with this problem without consulting any more physicians for 10 years.

Beginning in 2003, now a young adult, Danielle began seeking help from vascular doctors. She eventually had multiple difficult and painful procedures to try and remove the invasive venous malformation threading through the tissue in her foot. One procedure went too far, and, lacking proper blood flow, gangrene set in, requiring 9 months of wound care and loss of part of her toe.

These years of intervention left Danielle with a situation where much of the tissue in her foot is now scar tissue. She says the thing that saved her was graduate school; it kept her mind off of her difficult medical issues. She is now a published author of nonfiction books.

In early 2008, she started to experience severe and disabling depression, pain all over her body, and odd changes in her personality and behavior. The slightest thing overwhelmed her and she had no reserve for stress. She attributed these issues to the inevitable emotional stress in her life from having to endure many surgeries. She became humorless, irritable, and angry — while also developing severe pain in her arms, strange sensations in her chest and a significant tremor in her right hand. When she saw a neurologist in April 2009 about these symptoms, he dismissed her issues, suggesting that she get help from a psychiatrist. Along the way, she was diagnosed with chronic major depression, ADHD, fibromyalgia and carpal tunnel syndrome. Although she was treated for all of these conditions independently, nothing seemed to really help and her depression became disabling. She eventually withdrew from social interaction, fell into deep despair and, for the first time ever, contemplated ending her life. Only the support of her mother, niece and a few close friends kept her going.

Her local university was advertising for people with depression to participate in a clinical trial of transcranial magnetic stimulation and Danielle decided to give it a try, hoping that her depression might ease and she might then be able to cope better with her other problems. Part of the workup for this trial was an MRI. Oddly, they never called her to join the trial. Danielle followed up by asking why they never contacted her. The person on the other end of the phone said that there had been some non-specific changes in her MRI and that she ought to seek a neurologist.

Danielle was diagnosed with multiple sclerosis in May 2010. Her MRI showed 17 typical MS lesions as well as several lesions on her spine. Although she was diagnosed with relapsing remitting MS, Danielle suspected that she was probably progressive because she never had any identifiable relapse and her symptoms seemed to simply accumulate.

When she read about CCSVI online Danielle says she thought, "Now this is something that I can work with!" Knowing she already had another venous malformation, she felt this was likely to apply to her situation. Fortunately, compared to what she had been through with her foot, angioplasty sounded simple.

In mid–August 2010 Danielle became one of the first people to be treated in San Diego for Dr. Hubbard's IRB-approved trial. Her Haacke protocol report showing her flow quantification revealed that she had several narrowings in the azygous vein and problems in the upper and lower jugulars on both sides. She underwent a venous angioplasty in September 2010.

The interventional radiologist who performed her angioplasty discovered that she did indeed have two areas that required repair in the azygous vein, that both upper and lower jugulars required angioplasty, and also that the hemiazygous had a narrowed area that required treatment. Danielle had seven areas treated with angioplasty during her procedure. She had no complications and no discomfort.

Danielle underwent a second series of Haacke protocol diagnostics after her procedure. As with all patients in this IRB trial, there will be a very detailed report comparing her blood flow before and after the procedure, demonstrating any changes. Thus she will know how effective her procedure was at restoring blood flow.

This procedure has had a profound effect on Danielle's life. She says she did not feel different the first day, but the second day she felt lighter and free. The oppressive depression was almost completely gone and she experienced something that other patients have discussed online; she says it was like the world seemed physically brighter. Patients on TIMS who had treatment previously described this as if their vision became high-definition (HD).

A month after her procedure, Danielle says it's a relief to be free of the depression and to be herself again. She says she recognizes the woman in the mirror as the enthusiastic, excited and passionate person that she really is. Her family reports that she laughs and smiles and is her old self again. "You're back!" her niece announced to her one day. Danielle says that treatment was not difficult and if follow-up imaging at 6 months and one year with the Haacke imaging protocol reveals restenosis has occurred, she is prepared to have another treatment.

Summary

These two stories reflect the promise of very early treatment. While follow-up with this group was necessarily very short (at only four months and one month, respectively), the addition of very detailed flow quantification gave the interventional radiologist specific information about the efficiency of treatment with regard to blood flow in these individuals.

The nationwide IRB trial protocol prescribes follow-up flow quantification at six months and one year. Similar to the case with Dr. Campalani and his access to follow-up evaluation, these patients will have ongoing feedback about how well their bodies have maintained the angioplasty repair.

Stories on the Internet

It's easy to find stories on the Internet of people who have undergone an angioplasty treatment for CCSVI. Naturally, these stories are highly anecdotal, so bear in mind that such stories may not represent the whole picture. Chapter 8 describes several databases that hold links to some of these anecdotal accounts.

What follows are links to stories of two people who testified before the Canadian Parliament. These particular patient experiences may be of special interest because the circumstances lend more credence than typical anecdotal reports.

Steve Garvie testified before the Canadian Parliament about his CCSVI treatment on June 1, 2010. Mr. Garvie had been in an assisted living situation, but after his treatment became independent. His testimony can be heard at http://www.youtube.com/watch?v=KIs0JKOKX0A.

Liann Webb testified regarding positive effects of angioplasty for CCSVI before the Canadian Parliament on June 1, 2010. Her testimony is found at http://www.youtube.com/watch?v=hxUEOR5az9U.

8

Resources

We need answers and we need them now — posted on TIMS

The resources chosen for this chapter support the information presented in earlier chapters. It is not a comprehensive list.

Seeking a Trial

Presumably some people reading this book will be interested in participating in a trial. The following information will help accomplish this goal. Note: trials listed are those with available space for new registrants as of this writing. Please confirm the status of current trials with the FDA's site, http://clinicaltrials.gov.

Trials with Treatment

THE HUBBARD FOUNDATION • As mentioned in chapter 6, the Hubbard Foundation has established a nationwide IRB-approved trial that uses the Haacke imaging protocol (see appendix) to generate objective findings about how treatment affects blood flow in MS. This innovative trial is expected to be ongoing and other physicians with access to the right imaging equipment may enroll and participate in this trial at any time. The patients treated in this trial receive standardized imaging before and after treatment to evaluate how treatment impacted blood flow and MS lesions.

It is extremely important to understand that there is no prescribed angioplasty protocol for the interventional radiologist actually doing the procedure in this trial. The interventional radiologist participating in the trial will treat each patient on a case-by-case basis, doing his or her best to repair any venous malformations as they present. (Links to physician presentations are available later in this chapter so new physicians can benefit from pioneering physicians' experience.)

THE VASCULAR GROUP • The Vascular Group, in Albany, New York, is conducting a trial of CCSVI in MS, including treatment. The announcement of this trial is available at http://clinicaltrials.gov and the number of the trial is NCT01089686.

You can also search the FDA site for other ongoing and completed trials related to CCSVI. As of this writing there are only three trials listed, but since this is a growing area of interest more should be forthcoming in the future.

Trials with Assessment Alone

BNAC CTEVD TRIAL • Buffalo Neuroimaging Analysis Center began the CTEVD trial to investigate the prevalence of CCSVI in MS patients using MRV and duplex ultrasonography studies, as discussed in chapter 5. This trial is expected to continue over two years with several cohorts. People participating in the CTEVD trial do not get copies of their scans or data, and participation is at no cost to the patient. Information can be found at the BNAC webpage, http://www.bnac.net/?page_id=517.

BNAC also has a self-referral trial. In this trial participants pay for evaluation and the information is kept in a scientific database, but the patient is allowed to take the imaging scans to their local physician for evaluation. The Zamboni/Menegatti–style Dopplers have proven difficult to perform with reliable results, as discussed earlier in this book, but BNAC is one facility that has been trained by the Italian researchers themselves. The participating patient receives an MRI of the brain and neck, duplex ultrasonography, a one-hour visit with a neurologist, neuropsychological evaluation and a blood draw for a lab test. This gives people who may be receiving a procedure elsewhere an independent way to evaluate the effectiveness of such a procedure. Information is available at http://www.bnac.net/?page_id=626.

BNAC also has begun a small treatment trial called Prospective Randomized Endovascular therapy in Multiple Sclerosis (the "PREMISE" trial). Though recruiting is closed as of this writing, thirty people will be treated (http://www.buffalo.edu/news). Look for results in late 2011. If the findings of the first trial are promising, a larger trial will be undertaken.

Physician Presentations

The International Society for Neurovascular Disease, the ISNVD mentioned previously, is actively encouraging their physicians to share their experience with other physicians interested in the CCSVI model. The following sections provide links to physician presentations given by some members of the then-newly formed ISNVD at a symposium. Physicians interested in CCSVI are encouraged to contact the ISNVD for more detailed information and support. As their website comes online section by section, more information will be available for physicians (see http://www.isnvd.org/news/).

Brooklyn Symposium, July 26, 2010

The symposium held in Brooklyn gathered many of the physicians with the most experience with CCSVI to present their knowledge other interested physicians. These generous individuals traveled to this symposium at their own expense to share their experience with others. Although these presentations are available for patients to view, the information was geared toward the vascular doctors attending. Nonetheless, most patients will be able to appreciate and understand a good portion of the information offered. There are clickable links to these presentations on my website at http://CCSVIbook.com.

KEYNOTE SPEAKER, FABRIZIO SALVI, MD • Dr. Salvi is a neurologist working with the Zamboni research team. See Dr. Salvi here: http://www.youtube.com/watch?v=jlA2HrMHjNc.

SAL SCLAFANI, MD • Dr. Sclafani shares his experience with treating CCSVI. He talks about numerous issues related to treatment challenging practitioners. See Dr. Sclafani here: http://www.youtube.com/watch?v=puZO3W5gyIc.

GARY SISKIN, MD • Dr. Siskin shares his experience in treating people for CCSVI. He talks about the difficulties in treating these stenoses and insights his team has gained in their clinic. See Dr. Siskin here: http://www.youtube.com/watch?v=ZL5DmnXw9BQ.

DAVID HUBBARD, MD • Dr. Hubbard is a neurologist who currently has a national IRB trial to evaluate patients before and after CCSVI treatment using Dr. Haacke's protocol. Dr. Hubbard comments that MS is a disease of unknown origin. See Dr. Hubbard's remarks here: http://www.youtube.com/watch?v=FnQidgJbT1M.

TARIQ SINAN, MD • Dr. Sinan is a vascular doctor in Kuwait. His presentation focuses on techniques he and his colleagues have found helpful in their research. See Dr. Sinan's presentation here: http://www.youtube.com/watch?v=aLeRelZuUbE.

IVO PETROV, MD • Dr. Petrov, a vascular specialist from Bulgaria, presented his team's findings to date, reiterating that CCSVI is related to MS in the patients they evaluate. See Dr. Petrov here: http://www.youtube.com/watch?v=H2v8MIsyvhc.

Torrance Andrews, Seattle

Dr. Andrews is a fellow of the Society of Interventional Radiology, which means he is board-certified in the specialty. He is also a former chief of vascular interventional radiology at the University of Washington, and he has published many articles in his field.

He has expressed his personal opinion that patients with multiple sclerosis who wish to be evaluated and treated for CCSVI should have access to this assessment and treatment in their local communities rather than having to resort to medical tourism. He quips that if this is not a real disease, it is "a mass hysteria on a scale not seen since the Salem witch trials." See his presentation at http://www.youtube.com/watch?v=uAlbdW2aiYs.

Michael Dake

Dr. Dake gave a presentation about CCSVI at the Society of Interventional Radiology on March 14, 2010. This presentation explains the CCSVI theory in a balanced way and is a great introduction and overview for the newly interested physician. YouTube will automatically offer Part 2 as a related video: http://www.youtube.com/watch?v=adbVIRlh7h8.

Presentation by Dr. Haacke

Dr. Haacke gave a presentation explaining his protocol and how it relates to CCSVI treatment at a fundraiser in Detroit on August 7, 2010. The video is available here: http://www.youtube.com/watch?v=1fQckdv3vAc.

This video is understandable to laypeople and really makes it clear why, in Dr. Haacke's view, a patient might be interested in participating in this trial. If readers are considering asking a local IR to participate in a trial using this detailed imaging protocol, this video is good background to aid in the consideration.

Learning about CCSVI

Online learning ranges from poor sources to great ones. These are the author's preferred sources.

Fondazione Hilarescere

The charitable organization that supports Dr. Zamboni's work maintains a database of research related to CCSVI. Click on "publications" and all of the papers published by the Italian research team are available for free.

It's possible to read any of Dr. Zamboni's studies and print them out for practitioners whom you may wish to talk to about CCSVI treatment. This makes it very easy to help practitioners in your local community become familiar with this new paradigm. Many patients who have had success in securing a practitioner in their own communities have used these published papers in just this way. http://fondazionehilarescere.org

Online Database

There is an impressive database maintained online that includes not only links to papers favoring the CCSVI theory but also links to studies that are critical of CCSVI. Just click the "publications" link. This database also maintains links to blogs by physicians commenting on the subject of CCSVI (both positive and negative) and links to other presentations, news stories and clips that may be of interest to patients following the CCSVI story. Access this database here: http://csvi-ms.net/en.

National Institutes of Health

The National Institutes of Health keeps an extensive database of all published research called the National Library of Medicine. This database can be accessed online, and the name for the online access is PubMed. If a paper related to medical research has been published, it can almost always be located in PubMed.

The references for this book include the PubMed identification numbers (PMID). These were included specifically to make locating the information simple online. A PMID was available for almost every paper. In other cases, the references list a digital object identifier (DOI) when this was specified as the reference of choice by the authors of the paper. In that case, enter the DOI number into any search engine.

If you go to PubMed and enter the PMID into the search box, the abstract (a short summary) will come up immediately and there will also be a link to the whole paper. Sometimes the published paper is available for free; sometimes it must be purchased. To access PubMed go to http://www.ncbi.nlm.nih.gov/pubmed. You can also just ask your search engine (like Google) for "pubmed" and it will come up for you. PubMed is a fabulous resource.

Google Scholar

Google Scholar is one of my favorite search engines. This search engine only brings back scientific papers related to the search term; no advertisements and no news media stories. Also, if an entire citation (as opposed to just a summary or abstract) is free, Google Scholar denotes that by providing an additional link to the left of the main list of results.

See Google Scholar here: http://scholar.google.com/.

Get Connected with the CCSVI Community

Facebook

The Facebook page for CCSVI, *CCSVI in Multiple Sclerosis*, allows ongoing discussion among patients of all things related to CCSVI. Joan Beal, wife of the first patient treated for CCSVI in the United States, started this Facebook page so patients would have a place to meet and discuss their concerns and thoughts about the new model.

Joan regularly posts very thoughtful essays full of insight regarding CCSVI. Her topics range from the politics affecting the development of CCSVI treatment to clear explanations of the anatomy and physiology of the condition.

Activist patients are quick to post any new information related to CCSVI on this Facebook page. New studies, criticisms, governmental actions, and any other information related to CCSVI are offered for discussion.

See this page here: http://www.facebook.com/home.php?#!/pages-/CCSVI-in-Multiple-Sclerosis/110796282297.

TIMS

This Isms.com (TIMS), described in chapter 1, is considered the birthplace of the patient movement regarding the evaluation and treatment of CCSVI in MS patients.

The TIMS forum for discussion of CCSVI is populated not only by advocates of the CCSVI model but also a healthy number of skeptics who enjoy discussion focused on criticism of the model. Discussions can get heated, but the forum focused on CCSVI is rapidly becoming the largest forum on the website (http://www.thisisms.com/forum-40.html).

Other forums on TIMS can be found by scrolling through the list of other subjects. For example, there is a forum for discussion on stem cell treatments and people regularly post about stem cell approaches that do not include chemotherapy and radiation; in other words, they discuss stem cells for regeneration of damaged nerves. Some patients might find this of interest, particularly if they are very progressed.

Wheelchair Kamikaze

Marc, a long-time member of TIMS, started a fascinating blog about his experiences as a primary progressive MS patient. His balanced, thoughtful blog posts about CCSVI are widely appreciated. When the discussion gets heated or hyperbolic on TIMS, Marc is often the voice of balance and reason.

Marc had evaluation for CCSVI, but his issue was deemed untreatable with current techniques. That story is available on the following blog: http://www.wheelchairkamikaze.com.

Supporting CCSVI Research

Unlike most MS treatments that have been introduced in the past, treatments related to correcting CCSVI do not have a commercial driver. Unfortunately, the NMSS has proven reluctant to provide the kind of funding necessary to really understand the relationship between CCSVI and multiple sclerosis. As an example, BNAC researchers estimate they need $5 million to fund their CCSVI trials. The NMSS offered seven grants of roughly $700,000 each in June 2010 (NMSS 2010) and notably did not grant any of that money to BNAC.

As a result, patients have come up with innovative ways of supporting the needed research.

BNAC and MStery Parties

Interested individuals have the opportunity to help BNAC in raising funds for research of CCSVI through the methods discussed in this section. In fact, Dr. Zivadinov has commented that nearly all of the funds they've had available for their CTEVD studies have been raised by patients (Zivadinov 2010).

One very innovative way that BNAC made the experimental protocol available was to allow patients to travel to their facilities and get the full Zamboni protocol for a set fee. They called this program the CCSVI Database Self-Referral Program (see section on trials for more information).

Another novel concept is that of the MStery parties. This is somewhat like a sophisticated bake sale; a MStery party is hosted in your own community and the funds raised are sent directly to BNAC.

In my local community, a restaurant owner agreed to host a party for the cost of the food. The employees donated their time for that evening. The $100-a-plate dinner was fabulous, and Dr. Zivadinov made a speech via Skype regarding their progress in the research. This party raised roughly $15,000 for research. People across the MS spectrum attended this party. Attendees ranged from people who appeared able-bodied all the way to people who were at the far end of disability.

Individuals interested in attending or contributing to someone else's party rather than hosting their own can browse a list of parties in local communities on the BNAC website.

See BNAC's website with all the information about MStery parties here: http://msterypartyccsvi.bnac.net/.

Donations can also be mailed to BNAC at this address:

UB Foundation, Inc.
PO Box 730
Buffalo, NY 14226–0730

MS Innovations Fund

Holly Shean is the MS patient who suffered a hemorrhagic stroke after she was treated for CCSVI at Stanford. Holly was very disabled and the opportunity to be evaluated and treated for CCSVI meant a lot to her in spite of the fact that the treatment was very new and untested in MS patients. Her loss was a blow to the online patient community. Holly, who went by the online handle "Peekaboo," was a staunch advocate for the notion that people who had no options should have the opportunity to choose CCSVI treatment.

Because Holly felt so strongly about this, her family established a trust at Stanford in her name to support CCSVI research. Donations support preclinical research. As of this writing, the first paper on animals with occluded veins that was supported in part by this fund is about to be published.

Donations can be sent to the following address (specify that it is for Michael Dake's Innovations Fund):

Stanford University
Office of Development, Gift Processing
326 Galvez Street
Stanford, CA 94305–6105

Charitable Organizations and Foundations Supporting CCSVI

CCSVI Alliance

CCSVI Alliance is a 501(3)(c) charity begun by some of the first patients in America to be treated with angioplasty to alleviate CCSVI. Having the 501(3)(c) status identifies this organization as a legal and legitimate charity. It takes many months to get this kind of legal work done, and not all organizations claiming to be charitable have done this.

Members of the executive board and the patient board of CCSVI Alliance are either MS patients themselves or they are relatives that advocate for a family member who has MS. As of this writing, this organization is an all-volunteer effort. In the interest of full disclosure, I am on the patient board of this charitable group.

This charity was begun with the express purpose of advocating for patients who have CCSVI, providing a trustworthy venue for collecting donations intended for research, and disseminating accurate information to physicians and patients about CCSVI. Here is an excerpt from their website's homepage:

> Our aim is to provide MS patients, caregivers, and medical professionals with a definitive resource for learning [more] about CCSVI — the science, the process, and the patient experience. As more research emerges, replacing mysteries with data and speculations with fact, we will be here, objective and clear. Opening veins, opening minds. Let's get started!

One of the most informative sections on the website is the patient perspective section, which relates stories and anecdotes contributed by MS patients. As in this book, not all the stories are positive. This reflects a balanced perspective on what MS patients might expect should they undertake treatment.

As mentioned, CCSVI Alliance collects donations for CCSVI research. Although members of this charity do not conduct research, they work in close contact with the physicians doing the research mentioned in this book and are able to make informed decisions about where to send donations and institutions where they can make the biggest impact.

To access this site go to http://www.ccsvialliance.org.

Hubbard Foundation

David Hubbard, MD, the founder of the Hubbard Foundation, has an interesting story pertinent to the CCSVI movement (see his son's account of

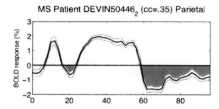
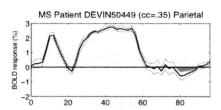

This BOLD image compares the brain oxygen levels before and after angioplasty. The image on the left taken before angioplasty shows a marked venous undershoot (the shaded area) that does not correct even by 90 seconds. After a local interventional radiologist performed angioplasty for CCSVI, the scan was redone with the results on the right. The reading on the right clearly shows values that have returned to normal: the scan reveals a limited venous undershoot that quickly corrects as it does in normal people.

CCSVI in chapter 7). As a neurologist Dr. Hubbard conducted a nationwide IRB-approved trial on a pharmaceutical in the 1990s. After retiring from his medical practice, he decided to establish a foundation with the goal of publishing research related to the brain and consciousness. As part of the research he bought a 3 Tesla MRI and began doing functional MRI in order to investigate this fascinating area of brain function.

When his son, Devin, was diagnosed with multiple sclerosis in 2009, Dr. Hubbard quickly brought himself up to date on all the things that had been learned about MS in the years since his residency. He was shocked to discover that although a number of pharmaceuticals were now available, researchers had only a vague idea of how these drugs worked and no certain knowledge of whether it influenced the long-term progression of the disease. When he reviewed the literature specifically related to autoimmunity, he was surprised to see that there was no solid proof that MS is an abnormal immune response and not just normal immune system activity reacting to some type of degeneration or damage (Hubbard 2010). All the big questions about multiple sclerosis remained unanswered.

Meanwhile, his wife, Arlene, came across patient information about CCSVI online. They decided that their access to the 3 Tesla MRI through the Hubbard Foundation was an opportunity to evaluate the new theory objectively.

Devin was evaluated in their 3 Tesla scanner using BOLD technology to quantify the oxygen levels in his brain. It was immediately apparent that his blood flow was poor.

The way BOLD technology works is that a person in the MRI machine is asked to look at two clocks, one with the wrong time and one that is correct. The patient is then asked to state the correct time and also click a button to select the clock with the wrong time. This demands several kinds of brain function to do it correctly, and the brain thereby uses oxygen to perform this complex set of instructions.

In a healthy person, there is a slight dip below the midline called a venous undershoot that quickly corrects after the mental activity. In Devin there was a large venous undershoot that took a very long time to return to baseline, indicating poor blood flow and poor oxygenation.

Dr. Hubbard was one of the first people to have an IRB-approved trial to evaluate angioplasty for CCSVI in MS patients using the Haacke imaging protocol and BOLD. In September 2010, the nationwide IRB trial was unconditionally approved.

Although BOLD technology is not new, using it to evaluate blood flow in CCSVI is a new application. Therefore, although patients do receive a BOLD evaluation as part of this IRB trial, that information is not part of their patient report because it is part of the research that's being done.

However, all the information obtained through the Haacke imaging protocol about flow quantification is available to the patient in a patient report (see appendix) when their doctor participates in the IRB trial. What this means is that an interventional radiologist in your own community can join this trial as long as he is able to do the specified protocol and gather the same data.

Dr. Hubbard and Dr. Haacke are working together. Scans from clinics participating in Dr. Hubbard's IRB trial will go to Dr. Haacke, who will objectively evaluate the scan results. Results are then entered in a registry to form a huge database.

For more information, contact Alexandra Hubbard (hubbardfoundation@gmail.com). To participate in this project, have any local IR who is interested in participating contact the above address with his contact numbers and address, and Alexandra will get back to him.

The Magnetic Resonance Institute for Biomedical Research (MRI Institute)

Dr. Haacke is the founder of the MRI Institute, a 501(3)(c) charity. Dr. Haacke has been mentioned many times in this book; for a short synopsis of his background, see the foreword of this book. The mission statement of the MRI Institute for Biomedical Research is as follows:

The corporation is formed to advance the basic science of magnetic resonance, and similar methods, its application to medical diagnostic imaging, the dissemination of the scientific knowledge thus obtained, and the furthering of public knowledge in the field of magnetic resonance imaging. Specifically, the purposes shall include the following:

- basic research in magnetic resonance imaging (and related fields) in a broad way so the results might apply to a variety of fields including medicine, biology, physics, chemistry and engineering;
- dissemination of the results of such biomedical research through publications, lectures, and other presentations;
- the training of scientists in the field of magnetic resonance imaging through internships, postdoctoral fellowships, lectures and other activities that might be associated with teaching institutions; and
- the promotion of general scientific education at all levels by participation in workshops, science fairs and other available mechanisms.

Tax-deductible contributions may be made at the site for support of Dr. Haacke's work.

To see Dr. Haacke's website and browse his material, including incredible pictures of the venous system in the brain, please go to www.ms-mri.com and www.mrimaging.com as well.

Note that Dr. Haacke is identifying those facilities that are using his protocol by showing a map with their locations on his website. As new facilities are added to his list of "centers of excellence" they will appear online. This will be a handy way to look for local facilities participating in this imaging http://www.ms-mri.com/ccsvicollaborator.php.

Foundazione Hilarescere

A foundation was established in Italy to support Dr. Zamboni's groundbreaking work. This organization raises donations, organizes fundraisers and engages in political advocacy, and it maintains the website that holds extensive information about Dr. Zamboni's work. All of the complete research papers done by the Italian research team are available on that website.

Contact the foundation or browse their information, which includes amazing pictures of venous malformations seen with venograms, at http://www.Fondazionehilarescere.org.

Direct-MS

Direct-MS is the second-largest charity in Canada advocating for multiple sclerosis patients. This charity was founded by Ashton Embry, PhD, when his son was diagnosed with multiple sclerosis.

An interesting feature of Direct-MS is that all the people on the board must either have multiple sclerosis or be the family member of someone with MS. There are no people with other agendas or potential conflicts of interest permitted on any of their boards and they don't accept any support from pharmaceutical companies.

Direct-MS funded the first trial on vitamin D and multiple sclerosis (Embry et al. 2000) at a time when the standard recommendation for vitamin D of 400 international units was considered adequate; this paper noted that relapses occurred when vitamin D levels were lowest, suggesting year-round supplementation at the 3,000–4,000 IU level may be desirable. This organization's advocacy for MS patients has always been ahead of the curve.

Dr. Embry's outspoken advocacy for treatment of CCSVI has attracted critics in recent years. The main complaint lodged by the critics is that he is not a medical doctor and therefore should not be speaking out on the treatment of patients. Yet it might be argued that the PhD, as a scientific degree, gives the laureate an understanding of research methods and statistics not held by the average medical doctor, whose curriculum does not typically include this kind of education. Dr. Embry has been an outspoken critic of neurologist obstructionism related to research of CCSVI (Embry 2010b; see also 2010c). Direct-MS has also made a generous amount of their donated funds available to study CCSVI.

The Direct-MS website is http://www.Direct-MS.org.

Plain-Language Summary

The research related to the CCSVI model has moved at an astonishing pace. Dr. Zamboni's third duplex ultrasonography study (the one with venograms) was released in December 2008. The speed with which this new paradigm has taken hold has left some people wondering what happened (Carlson 2010).

In reality, patient activism has pushed this research forward independent of traditional mechanisms of scientific inquiry. Patients and their advocates interested in CCSVI have made themselves available to support research on all levels, from funding trials to political advocacy, so that this new model can go forward with the speed its premise demands.

There are many people who find themselves becoming very busy as part of this patient activist movement, from Joan Beal, whose activities online to support her husband evolved into an administrative role at CCSVI Alliance and also administrative duties at the CCSVI page on Facebook, to Sharon Richardson, a person with MS and retired CFO who suddenly found herself president of CCSVI Alliance, to MS patients stepping up to the funding plate by hosting parties to raise research funds, recognizing that the only way this can ever happen is if patients make it happen, to all the CCSVI researchers who find themselves defending their work, sometimes against strident opposition, while simultaneously designing new studies or traveling a continent away to speak to government leaders about the need for advancing research into CCSVI.

It really is, as Dr. Haacke phrases it, a worldwide emergency; fortunately, patients have found ways to work around reluctant parties so the work can go forward immediately. No matter what the final analysis is regarding how MS and CCSVI interact, patients deserve the fastest possible answers. Nothing less is acceptable.

Appendix

Understanding the Haacke Imaging Protocol Report

If you are considering participating in a trial that uses the Haacke imaging protocol, or if you have had the imaging protocol and wonder what all the images in your report mean, the following explanation, written by Dr. Haacke, will be helpful.

MR Imaging with the CCSVI or Haacke Protocol

Reports from the Haacke protocol are often made available to the patients. The report consists of four major components:

1. anatomical images of major neck and brain vessels as well as the azygous vein;
2. flow quantification of major neck vessels, major brain dural venous sinuses and the azygous vein;
3. conventional anatomical MRI sequences showing brain structures and, when present, examples of MS lesions;
4. susceptibility weighted imaging (SWI) showing the small venous structure of the brain and iron lesions in the white matter, and measuring iron content in the major deep grey matter nuclei.

Basic Information

This section contains the demographic information of the patient, the institution where the MRI scan took place, whether the patient has received the complete CCSVI MRI protocol and, if not, what MRI sequences the patient's data includes.

Anatomical Information

In this section, two MRI sequences are used to evaluate the anatomical information of the major neck vessels and azygous vein. One is called 3D dynamic contrast-enhanced (CE) MRV or TRICKs; the other is 2D time-of-flight (TOF) MRV.

In the 3D CE MRV sequence, a contrast agent is injected into the right or left medial cubital vein (inside the elbow) through a power injector. While the contrast agent passes through the major neck arteries, brain arteries, brain capillary system, brain venous system and major neck veins, the MRI scanner takes snapshots (images acquired every 5 to 15 seconds) of the head and neck at different time points continuously for several minutes until most of the contrast agent washes out of the vascular system (or reaches equilibrium in the body).

Each snapshot consists of a 3D slab containing as many as 96 images (a set of very thin slices covering the head and neck). Each group of images is given a series number. All series contain the same number of slices and cover the neck coronally from the anterior to posterior where the major vessels reside. This method is used to show the anatomy of the vessels and, in particular, whether the major veins are present or not. As long as the contrast agent can go through, regardless of the blood flow's speed, the vessels will be seen in this set of images.

The first set of images in this section is composed of three images that are chosen to represent the arterial phase, the early venous phase and then a late venous phase. The arterial phase will only show the major arteries, including common carotid arteries, internal carotid arteries, vertebral arteries and major cerebral arteries. This method has been used in clinics for many years to image disease on the arterial side, such as artherosclerosis and stenoses of the arteries. Usually the later phases were discarded since the venous side was not considered as relevant.

The early venous phase shows the major cerebral sinuses and large neck veins with fast flow, such as the normal healthy internal jugular veins and subclavian veins. The later venous phase tends to show veins with very slow flow, such as the subcutaneous veins (external jugular veins) and the vertebral venous plexus. For the vertebral venous system or external jugular veins, depending on how large the vein is or how fast the flow is in that vessel, it can show up in the early venous phase or later venous phase. For instance, some MS patients develop very large vertebral veins; they can show up even earlier than the stenosed internal jugular veins. When the veins are shown, the arteries are still bright. This overlapping of arteries and veins makes it difficult to show veins clearly. In order to eliminate arteries, we do a subtraction of the arterial phase from the venous phase of interest. After this process, a set of subtracted images with veins only is generated. It is crucial to acquire high-quality arterial images in order to obtain good venous-only images.

Since the snapshot is acquired in a 3D slab, we can do a projection from any angle to get the best view of the narrowest part of the vessel. These images are referred to as the 3D rotation of the subtracted images, which comprises the second set of images in this section. In this picture, the existence, caliber, stenosis, and connection with other venous systems related to the internal jugular veins are discussed. Generally, colored arrows point to areas of interest on the images to demarcate individual vessels or abnormal areas. The third set of images focuses on the vertebral venous system, usually including three images; one is the whole slab showing the entire vertebral venous system which is followed by two images with a thinner projection. The goal is to show the vertebral veins and deep cervical veins separately. Depending on which phase shows the strongest vertebral venous signal, an early or late venous phase is chosen as the first image. The thinner slab is usually from the same series, but we choose the slices encompassing only the vertebral venous system to avoid overlapping with the internal jugular veins. In summary, the first three sets of images from our report are from 3D CE MRV data. The first set of pictures shows the dynamic changes of contrast agent going through the vascular system, the second set of pictures shows the internal jugular veins and the third set of pictures shows the vertebral venous system.

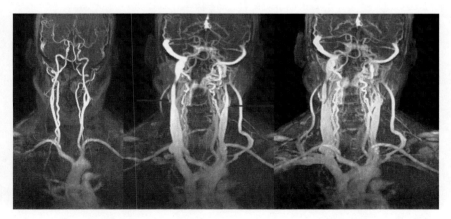

There are three images in the first set that look something like this one in the patient report. The left-hand image shows the arterial phase where the carotid arteries and vertebral arteries are clearly seen. The middle image shows the jugulars entering the image (the right internal jugular shows a bulbous structure at the bottom) and the left external jugular can be seen as well. The right-hand image shows more of the late phase, where the vertebral plexus usually becomes more visible.

2D TOF MRV does not require a contrast agent. The contrast is attained through suppression of the stationary tissue signal in the 2D slice and enhancement of the inflowing blood signal (also referred to as the time-of-flight effect). The arterial system is also purposely suppressed as described below so the vessels that are seen will be veins only. Since the blood is constantly moving, part or all of the saturated blood moves out of the 2D imaging slice and is replaced with fresh blood (not saturated) that is flowing into the imaging slice. Thus the signal from the blood vessels will be much higher than the stationary tissue. If we are only interested in the venous flow, then we can add another saturation pulse under the imaging slice toward the heart, which will saturate all the arterial blood that will be flowing into the slice. This way, only the venous blood gets refreshed with unsaturated blood. The result is a 2D TOF MRV image with high signal in veins and low signal in both arteries and stationary tissues. For efficiency purposes, the 3D CE MRV is usually acquired in the coronal orientation view in order to cover a larger region in a short time period. However, the 2D TOF MRV is best acquired in a transverse (sometimes called axial view) that is perpendicular to the direction of flow in the major neck vessels in order to get the best venous signal.

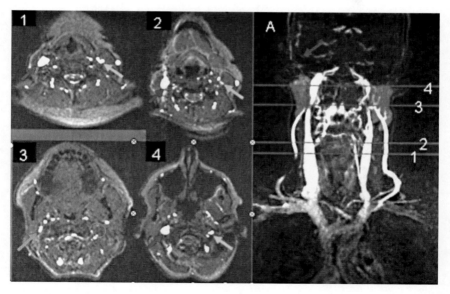

A comparison of the transverse images at different locations along the neck to view the cross-sectional vessel information. In the patient report this has colorful arrows indicating areas of interest. In the third slice, the left internal jugular cross-section disappears. Generally these transverse 2D TOF images are useful to quantify how stenosed a vessel has become.

So 3D CE MRV shows one whole vessel in the coronal projection, while 2D TOF shows only a cross-section of the vessel at different levels. This makes 2D TOF MRV complementary to the 3D CE MRV. Also, the in-plane resolution of the 2D TOF is four times higher than the equivalent reformatted 3D CE MRV view in the same place. In summary, the 3D CE MRV helps to localize where the abnormalities take place and the 2D TOF MRV shows the cross-section of the stenosed region. In this view, we can then determine whether the cross-section looks normal, is pancaked or is uniformly stenosed. So the fourth set of images in this anatomic section consists of 3 to 5 different slices showing the cross-section of the neck vessels at different levels.

We tend to choose the slices where the narrowest caliber of the vessel or pancaking takes place and the slices below and above the stenosis with normal caliber so that the changes of the vessel diameter can be observed from these sequential, but not continuous, slices from the lower to the upper level of the neck. The 3D CE MRV image is used as reference; the localization of each slice from 2D TOF MRV is marked as a red line (numbered) on the reference image. In this way, we have a good idea where the cross-section of the vessel from the 2D TOF MRV located. Another complementary piece of information that can be derived from the 2D TOF MRV is an indirect assessment of the flow information. Usually findings from 2D MRV agree with those of 3D CE MRV. When there is disagreement, both methods are compared. For example, when 3D CE MRV shows the vessel is present, while there is no signal from the 2D TOF MRV, this indicates that the flow speed is very slow and that the signal inside the vessel is saturated in the 2D TOF MRV just the same as the background tissue. When there is inhomogeneous signal inside the vessel, it usually indicates unsteady or non-uniform flow (this could be turbulent or vortex flow).

The fifth set of images in this section represents the anatomical information of the azygous vein. Most sites that use the CCSVI protocol use the 2D TOF method to image the azygous vein. The cross-section of azygous vein is shown on multiple continuous slices; we choose the slices that best show narrowing or pinching and also some slices above and below the narrowing with normal caliber. The transverse 2D TOF data is then reformatted to a sagittal view where the azygous vein can be shown in one single slice to see if there is a general narrowing trend. This data is often hampered by breathing artifacts so the best images are the transverse images. Owing to the breathing artifacts and some other technical limitations, the azygous vein is not always clearly seen even on the transverse view.

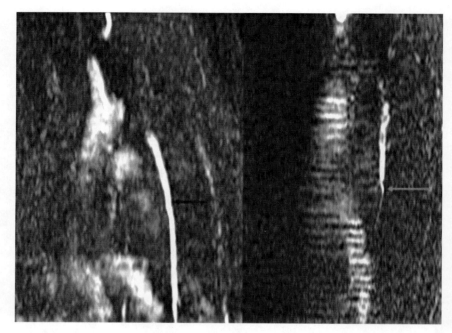

This image shows a normal azygous vein in the left and a stenosed azygous in the right image. Your patient report may show several transverse images as well, similar to what was shown in the previous figure. These are useful to look for pinching of the azygous.

Flow Information

Flow quantification is performed using a special MRI sequence by encoding the flow inside the blood vessels. This sequence generates two sets of images: a magnitude image and a phase image. The magnitude image shows the vessel anatomy and the phase image can be used to quantitatively measure the velocity and direction of the blood flow. The phase image contains the phase values of each voxel, which are proportional to the velocity of the blood flow at that voxel location. For a Siemens MRI scanner, if the phase appears dark this implies flow toward the heart. The darker the phase, the faster it flows toward the heart. If the phase appears bright, this implies flow toward the brain. The brighter the phase, the faster it flows toward the brain. If the data is from a GE scanner, dark means flow toward the brain, and bright means toward the heart. Dr. Haacke's group has developed their own software to process the flow data and to define a number of physiological flow measures to represent these findings.

First the user segments the vessels by drawing contours on the vessel boundaries. Then the software reads in the phase values inside each vessel contour. The software can decode the phase values to get the flow velocity of the blood flow through each voxel. Then the following parameters are calculated: integrated flow, volume flow rate, positive volume flow rate, negative volume flow rate, positive flow volume, average velocity, peak positive velocity, peak negative velocity, peak to average velocity ratio, average positive velocity and average negative velocity. The first five parameters have been chosen as most clinically relevant at this time, although many other measures are also available and stored for each patient.

Currently, most sites measure the flow at four different locations: (1) the upper neck level, (2) lower neck level, (3) straight and sagittal sinus, and (4) azygous vein. In each subsection (i.e., each anatomical region), the first set of flow images contains one magnitude image, 1 to 3 phase images, and an anatomical reference image showing where the flow quantification takes place. In the magnitude and phase images, major vessels are shown and indicated

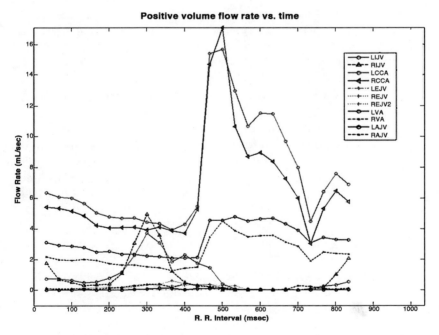

This is one of the many flow quantification graphs. The patient report shows arteries in red and veins in blue; this black-and-white version shows shades of gray. The lighter gray curves in the lower part of the image show the flow in the arteries toward the brain. The arterial flow peaks during systole around 500msec. The darker curves peaking around 300msec represent the flow in the veins going in the same direction as the arteries (the wrong direction for veins, i.e., reflux).

by colored arrows. Five graphs are shown, including total integrated flow per cardiac cycle; flow rates in the form of total, positive and negative; and average speed coinciding with the magnitude and phase images. These make it possible to determine if there are abnormal flow patterns such as no flow, reverse or reflux flow, and circulatory flow patterns (often the case for widened bulbous lower levels in the internal jugular veins). If the flow curves for a given vein fall through zero and change direction, then we refer to this as reflux flow. However, on occasion the vessel shows flow in both directions at any given time. This we refer to as circulatory flow.

The flow quantification at the upper neck level usually takes place at the second cervical vertebrae (C2). The lower neck level is at the sixth vertebrae (C6). These two different levels help us to get a feel for the flow coming immediately out of the brain and the flow at the lower level of the neck just above the confluence of the internal jugular veins with their corresponding subclavians before the blood goes back to the heart. The lower part is perhaps the most important because that is what represents most of the venous blood escaping from the entire head/neck system. The major vessels we can see for the neck include the internal jugular vein, common (internal) carotid artery, vertebral artery, vertebral vein, external jugular vein, anterior jugular vein, and deep cervical vein, as well as the anterior and posterior vertebral venous plexus. In some cases, we can only visualize some of the vessels, and in other cases we can see multiple vessels of the same name (such as two right external jugular veins).

This part of the report closes with a table of flow measurements both per cardiac cycle and translated into flow per second. Data are given for both the left and right sides separately. If there is much more blood flow in the arteries than the veins, this suggests that the vertebral plexus may be carrying that missing load. Azygous flow is also shown along with its own quantitative flow table.

Conventional Data

There are a number of conventional data sets that are collected. These include T1 weighted images (T1WI), T2 weighted images (T2WI), FLAIR (fluid attenuation inversion recovery) images and post-contrast T1WI images. These constitute part of the standard MRI protocol used to image MS patients clinically for many years. In this section, the first set of images represents the FLAIR data. FLAIR is very sensitive to MS lesions, which appear as hyperintense or hypointense signal in the white matter. We tend to choose 4 to 6 images at representative brain levels to show the MS lesions. The second series of images in this section is a comparison of the pre-contrast and post-contrast

T1WI. If lesions appear enhanced post-contrast, they are thought to represent acute lesions and these are then highlighted in the images with arrows.

Susceptibility Weighted Imaging Results

In this section, the first series of images is SWI phase images where lesions with high iron can be clearly seen. They can be MS lesions or hemorrhages. MS iron lesions can appear as a solid round, patchy dark, or ring-like dark signal inside the white matter. We tend to put the FLAIR images of the same brain level beside the SWI phase to compare the iron lesions on SWI and the hyper- or hypointense lesions on FLAIR image. For most cases, we can find corresponding lesions on FLAIR when iron lesions are visible, but not always. The second series of images in this section are MIPs of the SWI data where small venous structures of the brain, such as medullary veins, deep cerebral veins, and peripheral veins, can be shown. Dark areas representing iron in the basal ganglia are also shown. This set of images can tell whether the patient has diminished or engorged venous structures. The third series of images and plots represents iron quantification in the deep grey matter structures. There are seven structures in which we measure: (1) caudate nucleus (CN), (2) globus pallidus (GP), (3) putamen (PUT), (4) pulvinar thalamus (PT), (5) red nucleus (RN), (6) substantia niagra (SN), and (7) thalamus (THA). We have acquired SWI phase data on more than one hundred normal subjects. After measuring the iron content of the seven structures for each of the normal subjects, we have created a baseline of normal iron content in each nucleus. On the phase images from the MS patient, we draw the boundary of the structure of interest (usually following the contour of the nucleus). The software will generate the graph where data from the MS patient fits into the baseline graph. The region of interest (nucleus) is divided into two regions; one region includes those pixels with a phase value above a threshold value, which indicates high iron deposition (region II). The parameters we use include (1) average iron of the total region (TR-AI), (2) total iron of region II (RII-TI), (3) average iron of region II (RII-AI), and (4) normalized region II area (RII-NA).

In this section, the table contains a list of the seven structures and the four relevant iron measurement parameters. A check mark is placed in the box for that structure when there is abnormal iron content. If there is a check mark, the phase image and the graph will usually be shown. In this graph, the solid line is the regression line of the normal subjects. The outer dashed lines represent the 95 percent prediction intervals of the regression. We use the 95 percent prediction intervals to represent the normal iron deposition. Any patient beyond these intervals is assumed to have abnormal iron depo-

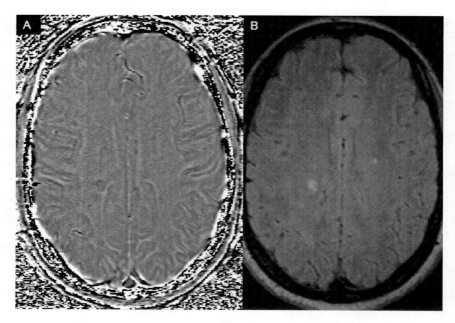

The FLAIR image (left) shows a number of lesions in this transverse slice. The SWI image (right) shows putative iron in one of the images in the right posterior portion of the brain matching the same large enhanced lesion in the FLAIR image.

sition in the structure plotted. The hollow square (left hemisphere) and triangle (right hemisphere) represent the measured result for the MS patient.

Why Is All This Important?

Having an MR scan prior to treatment is crucial for a number of reasons. First, it gives you a baseline of the brain tissue, MS lesions, vascular anatomy, flow characteristics, small veins, possibly perfusion (if that is eventually added to the protocol), iron content, and the presence of any microbleeds or thrombus. Apart from the critical issue of acting as a treatment planning guide for the interventional radiologist or vascular surgeon, this information is the baseline from which you can judge what happens in the future. For example, do lesions go away, does blood flow improve, and does iron content stay the same or reduce? Furthermore, if complications develop, this baseline scan can help determine where the problem lies. All this is not possible if you do not have the initial scan run with the CCSVI protocol.

Glossary

This glossary does not give all definitions for the words included
but rather the definition that applies to its use in this book.

AAN: American Academy of Neurology

Ablation: to eliminate or destroy. In stem cell transplants *ablation* usually refers to eliminating the bone marrow, which a stem cell transplant than rebuilds. This is done in leukemia to replace cancerous bone marrow and in autoimmune diseases to replace the immune system, which is generated in the bone marrow.

ACTH: adrenocorticotropic hormone

ADEM: acute disseminated encephalomyelitis (a temporary demyelination that sometimes happens after a viral illness or vaccination)

Acute: pertaining to a disease that is short-lived with marked symptoms, as opposed to chronic.

Adaptive immunity: immune system activity that comprises cells that are programmed or primed to attack targeted foreign antigens.

Adhesion molecule: a factor that causes white blood cells to adhere to blood vessel walls and migrate out of circulation into the tissue. Usually this factor is active when there are damaged cells or infection in the tissue. This is up-regulated in both CVD and MS

AHLE: acute hemorrhagic leukoencephalitis (a more aggressive version of ADEM)

Alemtuzmab: a monoclonal antibody still in trials that suppresses immune function (also used for cancer)

Angiogram, angiography: an invasive procedure for imaging the arteries with dye. The same process in veins is called venogram. "Angio-" refers to arteries.

Antibodies: immunoglobins that attach to foreign cells, marking them for destruction by the immune system. Complement attacks cells that are coated with antibodies, and the debris is cleaned up by phagocytes like macrophages (big eaters).

Antigen: proteins exhibited on the outside of cells that tell other cells what kind of cell it is

Apoptosis: programmed cell death. Ordinarily this is an orderly event in which old cells are systematically dissolved so new cells can replace them.

ASCT: autologous stem cell transplant

Atresia: absence or closure of a natural passage of the body

Atrophy: wasting away of tissue

Autoimmune: cells of the immune system targeting cells of the body. Low levels of autoimmunity are normal as part of healthy cell maintenance.

Axon, axonal: the long thin process of a nerve that extends out from the cell body conducting nerve signals to the next nerve

Azygous: vein that drains blood from the vertebral (spinal) system and delivers it to the superior vena cava, which attaches to the heart

B cells: cells of the adaptive immune system that make antibodies

Bidirectional flow: in reference to reflux this means blood flow going both directions

Biopsy: a sample of tissue removed from a living person. This is occasionally done in MS for atypical cases, but most of the time diagnosis is made on clinical grounds.

Blinded study, open study: in a blinded study either the physician or the patient do not know if they receive the placebo or the actual tested therapy. If it is double blinded, neither of them know. An open study is the opposite; everyone knows who received the treatment being studied.

Blockages: in this book this term refers to tissue blocking the vein and thus venous circulation. The words stenosis and occlusions are used interchangeably with blockages.

Blood-brain barrier (BBB): specialized tight-junction endothelial cells. Endothelium is the type of cell that makes up the walls of blood vessels; therefore the BBB is a specialized kind of blood vessel wall that has especially tight junctions.

BOLD: blood oxygen level dependent MRI (a kind of MRI reading that evaluates oxygen levels)

Budd-Chiari syndrome: a venous malformation in which a thin membrane has developed in the vein of the liver. In this disease there are fibrin cuffs around the vein and venous insufficiency in the liver, and the liver will fail if treatment is not successful. Treatment is removal of the membrane with angioplasty.

Catheter: a hollow tube for carrying fluid. The catheter used in a venogram is a very small double-lumen (two-channel) catheter that fits inside blood vessels and can deliver dye to the area of the venous system being examined, as well as balloons for angioplasty and other tiny reparative devices.

CCSVI: chronic cerebrospinal venous insufficiency

CD4, CD8: types of T cells

Centers of excellence: imaging facilities that Dr. Haacke recruited to participate in data collection using a very specific imaging protocol. The data gathered from the centers of excellence will be pooled in a worldwide registry so that researchers have access to and can analyze the information. Using information gathered in this database Dr. Haacke hopes to establish how treatment of blood flow abnormalities influences other findings obtainable using MRI, including iron stores, lesion loads, and flow quantification.

Chronic venous disease (CVD): poor venous drainage causing factors in the blood to leak out into the tissue. The result is iron in the tissue, immune system activity, and possibly lesions in the skin.

Chronic venous insufficiency (CVI): a blockage or problem in the vein causing a range of problems as a result of poor venous drainage (see chapter 4). This term is reserved for more severe venous disease in which actual lesions have developed.

cm H2O: centimeters of H2O (water). This measurement quantifies pressure; the amount of pressure in the area of the body evaluated displaces a column of water and this provides the reading. This is similar to a blood pressure cuff, which displaces mmHg (millimeters of mercury).

Cohort: one group in a study. There is usually a treatment cohort and a cohort that receives a placebo.

Collateral circulation: blood vessels that develop to take blood flow around an occluded area. These blood vessels cannot develop unless the occlusion is severe enough to cause changes in the immune system cells in the area.

Compartmentalization: the hypothesis that MS inflammatory factors get "locked in" behind the blood-brain barrier in areas where repeated MS attacks have taken place and these factors then damage tissue in a simmering inflammatory reaction, eventually resulting in secondary progression

Complement: an enzymatic protein that dissolves other cells. A phagocyte such as a macrophage cleans up the debris after the fact. Complement usually attacks cells coated with antibodies.

Control: a person in a trial who receives a fake drug or sham treatment for comparison to people who got the real treatment. This allows evaluation of the treatment in comparison to the placebo effect that the controls are presumed to experience.

CRAB drugs: this term collectively refers to the first-tier MS drugs: Copaxone (Teva), and the interferon drugs Rebif (Serono/Merck), Avonex (Biogen/Idec/Elan) and Betaseron (Bayer).

Cross-react: when an antibody reacts to a self antigen as well as the foreign antigen it was programmed or primed to attack

CSF: cerebrospinal fluid. This fluid bathes the brain and carries away some of the toxic by-products of metabolism. This fluid is constantly replaced and is exchanged roughly 4 times a day. This requires good circulation at the choroid plexus.

Cyclophosphamide: a drug originally used as chemotherapy and used today as an immunosuppressant in MS

Cytokines: factors in the immune system that turn on or regulate other immune system cells

DAVF: dural arteriovenous fistula, a pathological connection between an artery in the vein in the dura (lining in the central nervous system). This causes a knotty blood vessel that presses on spinal cord tissue, which results in symptoms similar to MS.

Dawson's fingers: lesions with a distinctive shapes seen on MRI that a radiologist recognizes as typical to MS

Degeneration: in relation to nerve tissue, this refers to loss of nerve cells

Demyelination: loss of myelin on the axons of the nerves, resulting in dysfunction

Deoxyhemoglobin: hemoglobin is the iron molecule attached to red blood cells that carries oxygen. One hemoglobin molecule can carry 4 oxygen molecules. After oxygen has been delivered to the cells using hemoglobin on RBCs, the hemoglobin is then deoxygenated (thus deoxyhemoglobin), and this form of iron is visible using SWI MRI. Thus deoxyhemoglobin can be used as an intrinsic contrast agent and is being used to elucidate the tissue perfusion in MS.

Diffusion: the process whereby particles dissolved in fluid move from an area of high concentration to an area of low concentration

Discovery: in reference to a new hypothesis, the process of learning about it. Researchers use observational study when discovery is the main goal.

Dissociation: not associated

DMD: disease-modifying drug

Doppler: shorthand term often used by patients in reference to an ultrasound exam that uses Doppler technology

Drop foot: a common problem in multiple sclerosis or other neurologic diseases in which the person cannot dorsiflex the foot (it tends to drag) when they walk, causing tripping

Duplex ultrasonography: a type of Doppler ultrasound that uses colorized technology to discern arteries from veins as well as a grayscale readout to evaluate the blood vessels

EAE: experimental autoimmune encephalomyelitis (the mouse model of multiple sclerosis)

EBV: Epstein-Barr virus, the germ that is responsible for a mononucleosis (also called glandular fever)

Efficacy: essentially effectiveness, meaning how well the approach in question works

Embolism: clot that blocks an artery or vein

Encephalomyelitis: inflammation of myelin in the brain

Endemic: natural to a given region

Endothelial dysfunction: the inability of endothelium to keep factors that belong in circulation from leaking out into the tissue

Endothelium: lining of the blood vessels formed by endothelial cells. The blood-brain barrier is a specialized type of endothelium with tight junctions

Epidemiology: study of the disease at the population level. Findings may or may not apply to individuals

Epiphenomenon: a side issue that occurs along with a disease but is not related to its cause. Researchers consider iron in the MS brain an epiphenomenon; they believe that iron is left over from nerve death and therefore not important

Evidence base: a term used to collectively refer to medical research published in peer-reviewed journals. Theories, ideas, and new models are not part of the evidence base

Excitotoxicity: when an agent that binds to a nerve cell to stimulate it causes its damage or death

Extracellular: around the cells (as opposed to inside them, which is intracellular)

Extracranial: outside the cranial area

Extravasated: leaked out. In this book, this typically refers to factors that belong in the circulation when they have extravasated into the tissue.

Ferritin: a cellular protein that stores and transports iron in a non-toxic form. See hemosiderin.

Fibrin: a fibrous protein that is the major component of a blood clot. Fibrin is deposited in areas that have been damaged.

Fibrin cuffs: cuffs that form around the veins in venous insufficiency. Among venous specialists, fibrin cuffs are considered a sign of venous insufficiency. There are fibrin cuffs in chronic venous disease, Budd-Chiari syndrome, and multiple sclerosis. Critics argue that fibrin cuffs are sometimes seen in areas of inflammation as well.

Findings: the results of a scientific study

First-tier drugs: in multiple sclerosis this includes the interferon drugs and glatiramer acetate; these are the drugs that are used first with the safest profile. Collectively referred to as the CRAB drugs, this acronym refers to the first letter of the brand names.

Fluoroscope: an X-ray–type device used in an operating room that takes a real-time picture of the blood vessels or other structures when the physician injects dye during an angiogram or venogram

Flush: in this book, related to drugs or supplements that cause dilation of the blood vessels and a flushed, red face as a result of dilated blood vessels

Germs: bacteria or viruses that can cause an infection. This term includes both of these infective agents and refers to them collectively.

Glatiramer acetate: a drug used for multiple sclerosis that is four amino acids linked together

Glia, glial: nerve cells

"Gold standard" test or exam: the test or exam thought to be the most accurate.

Gray matter: neural tissue (especially of the brain and spinal cord) that contains cell bodies as well as nerve fibers, has a brownish gray color, and forms most of the cortex and nuclei of the brain, the columns of the spinal cord, and the bodies of ganglia

Hemodynamics: the details of how blood flows in an area

Hemoglobin: a part of red blood cells that contains iron and allows red blood cells to carry oxygen molecules. Oxyhemoglobin is fully saturated with four oxygen molecules, and deoxyhemoglobin has surrendered its oxygen. Deoxyhemoglobin can be used as an endogenous (inside the body naturally) contrast agent and it is visible with SWI.

Hemosiderin: a degenerated form of iron usually created by macrophages when they are cleaning up red blood cells that have leaked out of circulation. Converting iron to hemosiderin denatures it so it is not toxic to nearby tissue, but it also no longer usable. The body can also sequester iron in the form of ferritin, though in that form it is not denatured.

Heterogeneous: of different types. Many people believe MS is a heterogenous disease because it presents in a heterogenous way (RRMS, PPMS, etc). The opposite is homogeneous, meaning all the same.

HFE mutation: altered genetics that result in different iron metabolism

Histology: a branch of anatomy that deals with the minute structure of animal and plant tissues as discernible with the microscope

Homeostasis: in balance. In people this means the systems are working in balance with one another in a person who is healthy.

Hypothesis: an idea that is not yet accepted as likely to be true; weaker than a *theory* (which is thought likely to be true), but the terms are often used interchangeably

Hypoxia: having low oxygen

Iatrogenic: caused by medical intervention

ICAM: intracellular adhesion molecule

Immune suppression, immunosuppressive: suppressing immune system function

Immune system: a variety of blood cells made by the bone marrow or lymph tissue for the purpose of monitoring the human body for problems that threaten health. Foreign tissue, germs, cancer, and old or degenerate cells are all managed by the immune system.

Immunoglobin: antibodies made by B cells, such as IgM or IgG

Immunological: related to the immune system

Immunology: the study of the immune system

Incidence: how often something occurs in a population

Indigenous: natural to the area

Infective agents: germs like viruses or bacteria collectively

Inflammation: a cascade of immune system activity that causes the affected area to be congested with fluid and immune system cells. If this occurs in a place where a person can see it, such as the skin, it will appear red and warm and will usually feel painful.

Inflammatory: a reaction that includes inflammation

Innate immune response: immune system activity carried out without primed or programmed cells. The most prominent innate response is phagocytosis, or scavenging by cells like macrophages (big eaters).

Integrin: an adhesion molecule

Intravascular: inside a blood vessel

Intravascular ultrasound: a tiny ultrasound device that is introduced through a catheter into a blood vessel to look at abnormalities

IRB: institutional review board. These review boards approve trials when they have met the standard of safety for the patients involved.

Iron: in this book, iron typically refers to that which is left over when cells die. Iron is an important part of red blood cells and makes it possible for them to carry oxygen. Nerve cells are cells that use a lot of oxygen and therefore also have iron in them. When either of these cells die, iron is left behind. Ferritin and hemosiderin are forms of iron.

Ischemia: tissue that is suffering from lack of oxygen

L hermitte's: common symptom in multiple sclerosis and some other diseases in which a person bends their neck and it causes an electric shock feeling

Laminar blood flow: blood flow that goes straight down the vessel in the intended direction

"Leaky" veins: simple term used here to describe increased diffusion of water molecules and other blood components across the endothelium

Lesion load, volume: the amount of MS lesions in a person's brain

Lipodermatosclerosis: hardening of the skin as a result of venous insufficiency

Lymphocytes: white blood cells such as T cells or B cells

Lymphopenia: low white blood cell counts (a common problem with drugs that suppress immune system function)

Macrophage: the largest phagocyte (also called "big eater"). Macrophages clean up debris left behind when other parts of the immune system have killed a target cell. Macrophages are also capable of scavenging on their own.

Magnetic resonance: the principle that guides magnetic resonance imaging (MRI)

Matrix metalloproteinases: these are factors that break down protein. MMPs are up regulated in both chronic venous insufficiency and multiple sclerosis.

Mean transit time: the length of time it takes blood to transit the brain

Memory: the ability of the immune system's B cells to remember a foreign antigen and attack it immediately on future encounters

Microglia: macrophages inside the blood-brain barrier

Micro-hemorrhage: local hemorrhage in tiny blood vessels to small to cause serious damage on their own

Migrate: in this book, referring to movement of immune system cells from the circulation out into the tissue

Mitoxantrone: an immunosuppressive drug

MMP9: matrix metalproteinases

Molecular mimicry: when a foreign antigen looks similar to a self antigen. This can result in cross-reaction.

Monoclonal antibody: an antibody made in a laboratory to target a specific cell

Monocyte: a type of white blood cell

Myelopathy: any disease or disorder of the spinal cord. Also may be used in reference to disease of the bone marrow.

NAA: n-acetyl aspartate (abundant in healthy brain tissue). MS patients have low levels of NAA even in normal-appearing white matter.

Nascent: beginning to develop

Natalizumab: a monoclonal antibody that is used in multiple sclerosis to stop the function of an adhesion molecule, preventing migration of inflammatory immune system cells into the brain.

Neural: pertaining to nerve tissue

Neurodegeneration: degeneration of nerve tissue

Neurotropic: helpful to the growth of nerve tissue

NMSS: National Multiple Sclerosis Society

Normal-appearing white matter: white matter that does not appear to be demyelinated or otherwise damaged but actually demonstrates low NAA levels

Objective: something that is identifiable by an observer. In contrast, subjective means something that only the subject can determine, such as how something feels.

Observational study: an unblinded study used when something new is still in the discovery phase, which allows the researcher to change his methods as he evaluates patients to reflect what was learned on earlier patients. This is a dynamic kind of study that evolves with what is learned.

Oligodendrocytes: cells in the brain that myelinate other cells

Open-label: a study in which everyone knows that they had treatment. There are no placebos as there are in blinded studies.

Opportunistic: an infection that takes advantage of the person who has immune deficiency or whose immune system has been suppressed. Healthy people do not succumb to opportunistic infections.

Outpatient procedure: a procedure that does not require admission to a hospital and an overnight stay. Typically people go home in a few hours.

Oxidative stress: physiological stress on the body that is caused by the cumulative damage done by free radicals inadequately neutralized by antioxidants. Free radicals can be created during natural biological processes. On a cellular level, oxidative stress is damaging to the cells.

Patent, patency: open, such as a vein that is not blocked

Pathognomic: unique to a particular disease. When a pathognomic symptom is noted, then the person has the associated disease.

Pathologic: pertaining to pathology, which means deviations from what is normally seen in a healthy person that characterize a disease

Peer-reviewed: research that was critiqued and approved by other specialists in the same field before publication

Peptides: factors made from proteins

Pericapillary: *peri-* means "around," and capillary is the term for the very smallest blood vessels

Peripheral immune cells: immune cells outside of the central nervous system. The blood-brain barrier forms the dividing line.

Perivascular: all around the blood vessels

Perivenous, perivenular: around the veins

PET scan: positron emission tomography (a type of scan that looks at a section of the body with different technology than an MRI, which is magnetic resonance imaging)

Phagocytes: a class of immune system cells, one of which is the macrophage, that play an important role in innate immunity as well as cleaning up dead or damaged cells that have been attacked by targeted immunity

Phagocytosis: when a phagocyte "eats" dead or damaged tissue

Phlebology: the European word for the study of the vascular system

Physiology: how the body functions (anatomy refers to its structure)

PML: progressive multifocal leukoencephalopathy, an opportunistic viral infection of the brain increasingly associated with suppressed immunity in multiple sclerosis

Presents, presentation: in relation to immune system function, this refers to one of the antigen-presenting cells, such as the macrophage, putting the "nametag" part of a foreign cell in their MHC II receptor. This primes the other cells of the immune system to attack that foreign cell.

Pressure gradient: in this book, pressure gradient refers to the difference in pressure inside the blood vessel when comparing pressure on both sides of any stenosis. The catheter that is used for the venogram has a device at the tip for taking pressure inside the blood vessel. As with the blood pressure taken in the doctor's office, the pressure is measured in mmHg or in cm H2O. Pressures inside the vessel are very low compared to arterial pressures taken with a blood pressure cuff.

Primed: this refers to the situation when an immune system cell is programmed to target a particular foreign antigen. This priming occurs when an antigen-presenting cell and helper T cells recognize a foreign antigen, then begin the immune system cascade that results in an adaptive immunity with T cells and B cells *primed* to attack the foreign antigen.

Progression, progressive: progression refers to accumulation of permanent disability. Progressive disease refers to a person with multiple sclerosis whose functional losses are continuous rather than remitting. Remissions suggest losses are due to demyelination whereas progressive losses are due to loss of nerves themselves.

Prospective: a study that enters people with the intention of evaluating a particular outcome in the future. This can be compared to a retrospective study in which people are questioned about something in the past. For example, to prospectively study lung cancer one might enter 100 smokers, then monitor them for four years to evaluate the number who develop cancer. In a retrospective study, 100 people with cancer might be asked questions like "how many packs a day did you smoke?" The prospective study is more reliable.

Proteinase: an enzyme that breaks down proteins. One example is matrix metalloproteinase, which breaks down tissue and is part of the problem in venous lesions in the legs.

RBC: red blood cells

RCT: randomized controlled trial

Reactive oxygen species (ROS): also called free radicals, these factors are the by-product of cellular processes and may damage neighboring cells if there are not enough antioxidants available to neutralize them

Relapse: sudden loss of function caused by inflammation and demyelination in the brain. Such losses of function frequently remit when inflammation recedes and an oligodendrocyte remyelinates the nerves.

Reflux: blood flow that is churning, chaotic, or flowing opposite the intended direction

Resistance index: a measure of how well blood flows in relation to breath. Dr. Zamboni's first ultrasound study utilized this exam.

Resorbtion: reabsorbing (in this book referring to cerebrospinal fluid). New CSF is made by the choroid plexus and the old fluid is resorbed so that overall the fluid is exchanged 4 times a day.

Restenosis, restenoses (pl): the re-narrowing of the vessel after it had been repaired using angioplasty or a stent

Retrospective: the opposite of prospective study. See prospective.

Scavenging: an innate immune system activity in which damaged cells are removed by phagocytes

Selection bias: choosing papers that support a particular point of view. Unconscious selection bias means the person does not make the biased selection intentionally and they are not aware that they are biased.

Self-limited: something that ends on its own without any intervention

Serum: the fluid part of the blood, as opposed to the red blood cells and white blood cells that are suspended in the serum

Shunted: in this book, shunted refers to blood that has been redirected out of its normal path to alternate blood vessels

Sonography: evaluating the structures inside the body with ultrasound

Standards of practice: the medical care considered standard within the specialty

Stem cell transplant: giving a person stem cells. This phrase may describe receiving stem cells after chemotherapy has killed the immune system (ASCT), or it may describe receiving stem cells for the purpose of repairing damaged areas (like brain cells damaged by MS). Note that such stem cells are usually harvested from the person before the chemotherapy.

Stenosis, stenoses (pl): an occlusion in a blood vessel that impairs blood flow

Subjective: symptoms that only the individual person can detect (such as feelings)

Suppressed, suppression: in reference to immune system suppression, this word refers to altering immune system function with a pharmaceutical so it is impaired and reduced. In autoimmune diseases these pharmaceuticals are thought to be helpful by reducing what is theorized to be overactive immune system function, though this approach results in suppression of all immune system activity so even natural immune activity is suppressed.

Surrogate markers: refers to features of a disease that are thought to be indicative of the disease process and have predictive value. In MS, inflammatory lesions and relapses are the widely accepted surrogate marker. Recent research has questioned the value of these surrogate markers since they are poorly related to progressive disease, and therefore have limited predictive value of this feature of MS.

T cells: these cells originate in the bone marrow and mature in the thymus; there are several types described in chapter 3, though the type most often referred to in MS is the myelin-reactive T cell, which has been programmed to attack myelin.

T helper cells: T cells that co-stimulate other cells of the immune system, such as antibody-making B cells

TCCS-ECD, or TCCD: terms used in Dr. Zamboni's research papers in reference to duplex ultrasonography

TGF-1: transforming growth factor I; this factor allows tissue to grow and thicken

Theory: an unproven idea accepted as likely to be true

Thoracic pump: the term that refers to the negative pressure generated in the thoracic cavity when a person takes a breath that likewise encourages venous return to the heart

TIMP-1: tissue inhibitor of metalloproteinases; this factor controls MMP9. Metalloproteinases break down tissue.

Transcranial window: a natural opening between bones of the head that allows a sonographer to view deeper tissue with ultrasound

Transcription: in reference to phosphatidylserine and the "I need assisted suicide" signal for the immune system, this means that the phosphatidylserine is reversed on the cell surface, which marks it as a cell that needs to be phagocytosed (eaten)

Transducer: the wand part of the ultrasound machine that is pressed gently against the skin

Ultrasonography: ultrasound

Ultrasound: a noninvasive evaluation using high-frequency sound waves that bounce off different structures inside the body in different ways producing a black-and-white image of those structures

Up-regulate, down-regulate: to activate or deactivate

Varicosities: distended veins caused by poor venous return

Vasodilators: substances that cause the blood vessels to temporarily dilate (widen)

VCAM: vascular cellular adhesion molecule, mentioned in relation to chronic venous disease. This is one of the adhesion molecules that makes it possible for things to migrate out of the circulation into the tissue.

VEGF: vascular endothelial growth factor; this stimulates the growth of new blood vessels, including the expansion of small vessels, so they may become collateral circles

Venogram: evaluating the vascular system by injecting dye into a vein, then looking at the vessels with an X-ray–type device called a fluoroscope that can see the dye. An angiogram is the same process in an artery.

Venous: pertaining to the venous half of the vascular system

Venous insufficiency: poor venous blood flow caused by an occlusion or other problem in the venous system

Venous ulcer: an open sore, usually in the lower leg, caused by venous insufficiency

Wallerian degeneration: degeneration of nerve cells referred to as "dying back" that occurs when there is damage to an axon and the area behind it dies. Traditional MS theory has offered that progressive MS is loss of nerves due to wallerian degeneration secondary to inflammation that happened earlier.

White blood cells (WBCs): lymhpocytes such as T cells and B cells

References

AAN (American Academy of Neurology). 2010. April 14: A live Web forum on CCSVI and what it could mean to people with MS. Transcript of live-stream forum.

Adams, C. 1988. "Perivascular iron deposition and other vascular damage in multiple sclerosis." *The Journal of Neurology, Neurosurgery and Psychiatry.* Feb;51:260–65. PMID:3346691.

Adhya, S., G. Johnson, J. Herbert, H. Jaggi, J.S. Babb, R.I. Grossman, and M. Inglese. 2006. "Pattern of hemodynamic impairment in multiple sclerosis: dynamic susceptibility contrast perfusion MR imaging at 3.0 T." *Journal of Neuroimaging.* Dec;33(4):1029–35. PMID:16996280.

Alguire P., and B. Mathes. 2007. "Chronic venous insufficiency and venous ulceration." *The Journal of General Internal Medicine.* Jun;12(6):374–83. PMID:9192256.

Allhorn, M., K. Lundqvist, A. Schmidtchen, and B. Akerstrom. 2003. "Heme scavenging role of a-one micro globulin in chronic ulcers." *The Journal of Investigational Dermatology.* Sep;121(3):640–46. PMID:12925227.

Al-Omari, M.H., L.A. Rousan. 2010. "Internal jugular vein morphology and hemodynamics in patients with multiple sclerosis." *International Angiology.* Apr; 29(2):115–20. PMID:20351667.

Andrews, T. 2010. CCSVI presentation for lecture series *Advances in Interventional Radiology.* Available online at http://www.youtube.com/watch?v=uAl bdW2aiYs (accessed September 3, 2010).

Angell, M. 2005. *The Truth About Drug Companies: How They Deceive Us and What to Do About It.* New York: Random House.

Angioplasty.org. http://www.ptca.org (accessed August 2010).

Arnon, R., and R. Aharoni. 2004. "Mechanism of action in glatiramer acetate and its potential for development in new applications." *Proceedings of the National Academy of Science USA.* Oct 5;101 Suppl 2:14593–98. PMID:15371592.

Bakshi, R., R. Benedict, R. Bermel, S. Caruthers, S. Puli, C. Tjoa, A. Fabiano, and L. Jacobs. 2002. "T2 Hypointensity in the deep grey matter of patients with multiple sclerosis." *Archives of Neurology.* Aug;59:62–68. PMID:17468444.

Barkhof, F. 1999. "MRI in multiple sclerosis: correlation with expanded disability scale (EDSS)." *Multiple Sclerosis.* Aug;5(4):283–86. PMID:10467389.

Barnett, M., A. Henderson, and J. Prineas. 2006. "The macrophage in MS: just a scavenger after all?" *Multiple Sclerosis.* Apr;12(2):121–32. PMID:16622941.

Barnett, M., J. Parratt, J. Pollard, and J.

Prineas. 2009a. "MS: is it one disease?" *International MS Journal.* Jun;16(2):57–65. PMID:19671369.

Barnett, M., J. Parratt, and J. Prineas. 2009b. "Multiple sclerosis: distribution of inflammatory cells in newly forming MS lesions." *Annals of Neurology.* Dec; 66:739–53. PMID:20035511.

Barnett, M., and J. Prineas. 2004. "Relapsing and remitting multiple sclerosis: pathology of the newly forming lesion." *Annals of Neurology.* Apr; 55(4):458–68. PMID:15048884.

Barnett, M., and I. Sutton. 2006. "The pathology of multiple sclerosis: a paradigm shift." *Current Opinion in Neurology.* Jun;19:242–47. PMID:1670282 9.

Bartolomei, I., F. Salvi, R. Galeotti, E. Salviato, M. Alcanterini, E. Menegatti, M. Mascalchi, and P. Zamboni. 2010. "Hemodynamic patterns of chronic cerebrospinal venous insufficiency in multiple sclerosis: correlation with symptoms at onset and clinical course." *International Angiology.* Apr;29(2): 183–88. PMID:20351674.

Beers, M., and R. Berkow (eds). *The Merck Manual Edition 17.* Whitehouse Station, NJ: Merck.

Behan, P., and A. Chaudhuri. 2005. "Looking beyond autoimmunity." *Journal of the Royal Society of Medicine.* Jul;98(7): 303–6. PMID:15994589.

Behan, P., and A. Chaudhuri. 2002. "The pathogenesis of multiple sclerosis revisited." *The Journal of the Royal College of Physicians of Edinburgh.* 32(4):244–65.

Bennett, M.H., and R. Heard. 2004. "Hyperbaric oxygen therapy for multiple sclerosis." *Cochrane Database of Systematic Reviews.* Issue 1. Art. No.: CD003057. DOI:10.1002/14651858. CD003057.pub2 (accessed June 15, 2010).

Berenson, R. 2010. "Implementing health care reform: why Medicare matters." *New England Journal of Medicine.* Available online at http://healthcarere form.nejm.org/?p=3480#printpreview (accessed June 14, 2010).

Bergan, J., G.W. Schmid-Schönbein, P.D. Smith, A.N. Nicolaides, M.R. Boisseau, and B. Eklof. 2006. "Chronic venous disease." *New England Journal of Medicine.* Aug3;355(5):488–98. PMID: 16885552.

Berger, J., and S. Houff. 2009. "Opportunistic infections and other risks with newer multiple sclerosis therapies." *Annals of Neurology.* Apr;65(4):367–77. PMID:19399841.

Berger, J., S. Sheremata, L. Resnick, S. Atherton, M. Fletcher, and M. Norenberg. 1989. "Multiple sclerosis like illness occurring with HIV infection." *Neurology.* Mar;39(3):324–29. PMID: 2927638.

Bitsch, A., J. Schuchardt, S. Bunkowski, T. Kuhlmann, and W. Bruck. 2000. "Acute axonal injury in multiple sclerosis correlation with demyelination and inflammation." *Brain.* Jun;123(6): 1174–83. PMID:10825356.

Bjartmer, C., and B. Trapp. 2001. "Axonal and neuronal degeneration in multiple sclerosis mechanisms and functional consequences." *Current Opinion in Neurology.* Jun;14(3):271–78. PMID: 11371748.

Blackwell, T. 2010. "Is new MS research the real thing or a media driven frenzy?" *National Post,* January 22, 2010. Available online at http://www.nationalpost. com (accessed January 23, 2010).

Boggild, M., J. Palace, P. Barton, Y. Ben-Shlomo, T. Bregenzer, C. Dobson, and R. Gray. 2009. "Multiple sclerosis risk sharing scheme: two year results of clinical cohort study with historical comparator." *British Medical Journal.* Dec 2;339:b4677. DOI:10.1136/bmj. b4677. PMID:19955128.

Bourgouin, P., D. Tampieri, D. Melancon, R. del Carpio, and R. Ethier. 1992. "Superficial siderosis of the brain following unexplained subarachnoid hemorrhage: MRI diagnosis and clinical significance." *Neuroradiology*. 34(5):407–10. PMID:1407522.

Bradley, W. 2008. "Idiopathic normal pressure hydrocephalus: new findings and thoughts on etiology." *American Journal of Radiology*. Jan;29:1–3. PMID: 18192342.

Bradley, W., D. Scalzo, J. Queralt, W. Nitz, D. Atkinson, and P. Wong. 1996. "Normal-pressure hydrocephalus: evaluation with cerebrospinal fluid flow measurements at MR imaging." *Radiology*. Feb;198(2):523–29. PMID:85 96861.

Brandes, L. 2010a. "CCSVI trials and tribulations: do we already know the answer to this question?" *CTV Mednews Express*, June 14, 2010. Available online at http://healthblog.ctv.ca/post/CCS VI-trials-and-tribulations-Do-we-al ready-know-the-answer-to-the-ques tion.aspx (accessed June 14, 2010).

Brandes, L. 2010b. "When studies disagree: cancer treatment and CCSVI as examples." *CTV Mednews Express*, June 21, 2010 (accessed August 1, 2010).

Breij, E., B. Brink, R. Veerhuis, C. van den Berg, R. Vloet, R. Yan, C. Dijkstra, P. van der Valk, and L. Bo. 2008. "Homogeneity of active demyelinating lesions in established multiple sclerosis." *Annals of Neurology*. Jan;63(1):16–25. PMID:18232012.

Brenner, S. 2009. E-letter comment on "Chronic cerebrospinal venous insufficiency," by Zamboni et al. Apr;80 (4):392–99. Available online at http://jnnp.bmj.com/content/80/4/392.long# responses (accessed June 17, 2009).

Brickner R. 1953. "Essential precautions in treatment of new phenomena in multiple sclerosis." *AMA Archives of Neurology and Psychiatry*. Oct;70(4): 483–88. PMID:13091497.

Brink, B., E. Breij, R. Veerhuis, P. van der Valk, C. Dijkstra, L. Bo. 2005. "The pathology of multiple sclerosis is location dependent: no significant complement activation in cortical lesions." *The Journal of Neuropathology and Experimental Neurology*. Feb;64(2):147–55. PMID:15751229.

Brinkman, D., C. Jol-van der Zijde, M. ten Dam, P. te Boekhorst, R. ten Cate, N. Wulffraat, R. Hintzen, J. Vossen, and M. van Tol. 2007. "Resetting the adaptive immune system after autologous stem cell transplantation: lessons from responses to vaccines." *The Journal of Clinical Immunology*. Nov;27 (6):647–58. PMID:17690955.

Brown, J. 2005. "The role of the fibrin cuff in the development of venous ulcer." *Journal of Wound Care*. Jul;14 (7):324–27. PMID:160448219.

Bruck, W. 2005. "Inflammatory demyelination is not central to the pathogenesis of multiple sclerosis." *The Journal of Neurology*. Nov;252(Suppl 5):v10–15. PMID:16254696.

Burgetova, A., Z. Siedl, J. Krasensky, D. Horakova, M. Vanekova. 2010. "Multiple sclerosis and the accumulation of iron in the basal ganglia: quantitative assessment of brain iron using MRI T2 relaxometry." *European Neurology*. 2010;63(3):136–43. PMID:20130410.

Burton, T. 2010. "Stanford MS program halted amid controversy." *The Wall Street Journal*. March 25, 2010.

Caillier, S., F. Briggs, B.A. Cree, S.E. Baranzini, M. Fernandez-Viña, P.P. Ramsay, O. Khan, W. Royal 3rd, S.L. Hauser, L.F. Barcellos, and J.R. Oksenberg. 2008. "Uncoupling the roles of HLA-DRB1 and HLA-DRB5 genes in multiple sclerosis." *The Journal of Immunology*. Oct 15;181(8):5473–80. PMID:18832704.

Cannella, B., S. Gaupp, K. Omari, and C. Raine. 2007. "Multiple sclerosis: death receptor expression and oligodendrocyte apoptosis in established lesions." *The Journal of Neuroimmunology.* Aug;188(1–2):128–37. PMID:176 10960.

Carlson, K. 2010. "Don't base MS cure on hope." *Montreal Gazette*, July 1, 2010.

Charlton, B. 2008. "False, trivial, obvious: why new and revolutionary theories are typically disrespected." *Medical Hypotheses.* 2008;71(1):1–3. PMID:18434041.

Cejas, C., L. Cisneros, R. Lagos, C. Zuk, and F. Ameriso. 2010. "Internal jugular vein in competence is highly prevalent in transient global amnesia." *Stroke.* Jan;41(1):67–71. PMID:19926838.

Chaudhuri, A. 2004. "Multiple sclerosis is not an autoimmune disease." Comment in *Archives of Neurology.* Oct;61 (10):1610–12. PMID:15477520.

Chu, A.B., J.L. Sever, D.L. Madden, M. Iivanainen, M. Leon, W. Wallen, B.R. Brooks, Y.J. Lee, and S. Houff. 1983. "Oligoclonal bands in cerebrospinal fluid in various neurological disease." *Annals of Neurology.* Apr;13(4):434–39. PMID:6838175.

Chu, S., S. Shyur, Y. Peng, C. Wu, C. Chang, C. Lai, and W. Wu. 2002. "Juvenile idiopathic arthritis with pulmonary hemosiderosis: a case report." *Journal of Microbiology, Immunology and Infection.* Jun;35(2):133–35. PMID: 12099336.

Cohen, B. 2004. *PTCA: a history.* Documentary. Venture Digital LLC.

Cohen, B. 2003. *Vascular pioneers: evolution of a specialty.* Documentary. Venture Digital LLC.

Cohen, B. 2010. "Three months of plavix after a stent: when less may be more." The Stent Blog on Angioplasty.org. Available online at http://www.ptca. org/voice/archives/2010_0311.html (accessed August 22, 2010).

Coles, A., D. Compston, K. Selmaj, et al. 2009. "Alemtuzumab vs interferon beta-1a in early multiple sclerosis and compassionate use." *The Journal of the Royal College of Physicians of Edinburgh.* 2009;39:35–37. Available online at http://www.rcpe.ac.uk/journal/issue/jo urnal_39_1/kelly.pdf (accessed August 17, 2010).

Coles, A., D. Compston, K. Selmaj, S. Lake, S. Moran, D. Margolin, P. Tandon, et al. 2008. "Alemtuzumab vs. interferon beta-1a in early multiple sclerosis." *New England Journal of Medicine.* Oct 23;359(17):1786–1801. PMID:189 41664.

Coles, A., A. Cox, E. Page, J. Jones, S. Trip, J. Deans, S. Seaman, D. Miller, G. Hale, H. Waldmann, and A. Compston. 2002. "The window of therapeutic opportunity in multiple sclerosis." *The Journal of Neurology.* Jan;253(1): 98–108. PMID:1604421.

Confavreux, C., and S. Vukusic. 2006a. "Accumulation of irreversible disability in multiple sclerosis: epidemiology to treatment." *Clinical Neurology and Neurosurgery.* Mar;108(3):327–32. PM ID:16413961.

Confavreux, C., and S. Vukusic. 2006b. "The natural history of multiple sclerosis." *La Revue du Practicien.* Jun 30;56(12):1313–20. PMID:16948219.

Confavreux, C., S. Vukusic, T. Moreau, and P. Adeleine. 2000. "Relapses and progression of disability in multiple sclerosis." *New England Journal of Medicine.* Nov 16;343(20):1430–38. PMID: 11078767.

Coo, H., and K.J. Aronson. 2004. "A systematic review of several potential nongenetic risk factors for multiple sclerosis." *Neuroepidemiology.* Jan–Apr;23 (1–2):1–12. PMID:14739563.

Corcoran, T. 2010. "A cure in sight? Not so fast." *National Post*, January 25, 2010. Available online at http://net

work.nationalpost.com/np/blogs/fp comment/archive/2010/01/25/terence-corcoran-a-cure-in-sight-not-so-fast. aspx (accessed August 18, 2010).

Coyle, P. 2006. "Management of suboptimal responders." Presentation October 12, 2006. Archived on Medscape in CME activity, *MS treatment: the importance of early intervention and comprehensive disease management.* http://www.medscape.com/viewprogram/6005 (accessed May 16, 2010).

Craelius, W., M.W. Migdal, C.P. Luessenhop, A. Sugar, and I. Mihalakis. 1982. "Iron deposits surrounding multiple sclerosis plaques." *Archives of* Pathology *& Laboratory* Medicine. Aug;106(8): 397–99. PMID:6896630.

Cregan, S., A. Fortin, J. MacLaurin, S. Callaghan, F. Cecconi, S. Yu, T. Dawson, V. Dawson, D. Park, G. Kroemer, and R. Slack. 2002. "Apoptosis-inducing factor is involved in the regulation of caspase-independent neuronal cell death." *The Journal of Cell Biology.* Aug 5;158(3):507–17. PMID:12147675.

CTV Winnipeg. 2010a. High rates of vein blockages found in MS patients. February 10, 2010. Available online at http://www.ctv.ca/CTVNews/TopStories/20100210/ccsvi_100210/ (accessed October 1, 2010).

CTV Winnipeg. 2010b. Agency aims to fund research into angioplasty for MS. June 15, 2010. Available online at http://winnipeg.ctv.ca/servlet/an/local/CTV News/20100615/ms-study-cihr-100615/20100615/?hub=WinnipegHome (accessed June 19, 2010).

Dake, M. 2010a. Presentation at the Society of Interventional Radiology annual meeting, March 14, 2010. Available online at http://www.youtube.com/watch?v=adbVIR1h7h8 (accessed August 29, 2010).

Dake, M. 2010b. Presentation at MSketeers fundraiser, August 16, 2010. Available online at http://www.youtube.com/watch?v=ocu7FURU8Bc (accessed August 27, 2010).

Dale, R., and J. Branson. 2005. "Acute disseminated encephalomyelitis or multiple sclerosis: can the initial presentation help in establishing a correct diagnosis?" *Archives of Disease in Childhood.* Jun;90(6):636–39. PMID:15908 633.

Dashkoff, N., G. Blessios, and M. Cox. 2010. "Migration of covered stents from hemodialysis A-V access to the pulmonary artery: percutaneous stent retrieval and procedural trends." Catheterization and cardiovascular interventions published online by Wiley Interscience. DOI:10.1002/ccd.22553 (accessed August 18, 2010).

Davidson, J. 1998. "Animal models for wound repair." *Archives of Dermatological Research.* 290(Suppl):s1–s11.

Deluca, G., K. Williams, G. Evangelou, G. Ebers, and M. Esiri. 2006. "The contribution of demyelination to axonal loss in multiple sclerosis." *Brain.* Jun;129(Part 6):1507–16. PMID:16597 651.

Doepp, F., P. Friedemann, J. Valdueza, K. Schmeirer, and S. Schreiber. 2010. "No cerebro-cervical venous congestion in patients with multiple sclerosis." *Annals of Neurology.* Aug;68(2):173–83. PMID: 20695010.

Dotter, C. 1964. *Transluminal Angioplasty.* Documentary. Available online at http://www.ptca.org/archive/bios/dotter.html (accessed August 20, 2010).

Eberhardt, R., and J. Raffetto. 2005. "Chronic venous insufficiency." *Circulation.* May 10;111(18):2398–2409. PM ID:15883226.

Ebers, G.C., L. Heigenhauser, M. Daumer, C. Lederer, and J.H. Noseworthy. 2008. "Disability as an outcome in MS clinical trials." *Neurology.* Aug 26;71 (9):624–31. PMID:18480462.

Ebers, G., A. Traboulsee, D. Li, D. Langdon, A. Reder, D. Goodin, T. Bogumil, K. Beckmann, C. Wolf, A. Konieczny. 2010. "Analysis of clinical outcomes according to original treatment groups 16 years after the pivotal IFNB-1b trial." *The Journal of Neurosurgery and Psychiatry.* Aug;81(8):907–12. PMID:2056 2430.

Einsten, O., Y. Friedman-Levi, N. Grigoriadis, and T. Ben-Hur. 2009. "Transplanted neural precursors enhance host brain-derived myelin regeneration." *The Journal of Neuroscience.* Dec 16;29 (50):15694–702. PMID:20016084.

Elward, K., M. Griffiths, M. Mizuno, C.L. Harris, J.W. Neal, B.P. Morgan, and P. Gasque. 2005. "CD46 plays a key role in tailoring innate immune recognition of apoptotic and necrotic cells." *Journal of Biological Chemistry.* Oct 28;280(43): 36342–54. PMID:16087667.

Embry, A. 2010a. "Integrating CCSVI and CNS autoimmunity in the disease model for MS." *International Angiology.* Apr;29(2):93–94. PMID:20351665.

Embry, A. 2010b. Letter to Parliamentarians. June 16, 2010. Available online at http://www.direct-ms.org/magazines/ Letter%20to%20Parliamentarians %2016%2006%2010.pdf (accessed June 17, 2010).

Embry, A. 2010c. "New studies show the MS drugs don't slow progression." July 7, 2010. Comment available online at http://www.direct-ms.org (accessed July 10, 2010).

Embry, A., L. Snowden, and R. Vieth. 2000. "Vitamin D and seasonal fluctuation of gadolinium enhancing magnetic resonance imaging lesions in multiple sclerosis." *Annals of Neurology.* Aug;48(2): 271–72. PMID:10939587.

Evans, E., H. Thornton, and I. Chalmers. 2006. *Testing treatments.* Originally published by The British Library, 2006; reprint Pinter & Martin, 2010.

Exley, C., G. Mamutse, O. Korchazhkina, E. Pye, S. Strekopytov, A. Polwart, and C. Hawkins. 2006. "Elevated urinary excretion of aluminum and iron in multiple sclerosis." *Multiple Sclerosis.* Oct;12(5):533–40. PMID:17086897.

Fainardi, E., M. Castellazzi, S. Seraceni, E. Granieri, and C. Contini. 2008. "Under the microscope: focus on Chlamydia pneumoniae infection and multiple sclerosis." *Current Neurovascular Research.* Feb;5(1):60–70. PMID:18289023.

Fainardi, E., M. Castellazzi, C. Tamborino, S. Seraceni, M.R. Tola, E. Granieri, and C. Contini. 2009. "Chlamydia pneumoniae-specific intrathecal oligoclonal antibody response is predominantly detected in a subset of multiple sclerosis patients with progressive forms." *Journal of Neuroviology.* Dec;15(5–6):425–33. PMID:20053141.

Farge, D., M. Labopin, A. Tyndall, A. Fassas, G. Mancardi, J. VanLaar, J. Ouyang, T. Kozak, J. Moore, I. Kotter, V. Chesnel, A. Marmont, A. Gratwohl, and R. Saccardi. 2010. "Autologous hematopoietic stem cell transplantation for autoimmune diseases: an observational study on 12 years' experience from the European Group for Blood and Marrow Transplantation Working Party on Autoimmune Diseases." *Haematologica.* Feb;95(2):284–92. PMID:19773265.

Fassas, A., and G. Mancardi. 2008. "Autologous hemopoietic stem cell transplantation for multiple sclerosis: is it worthwhile?" *Autoimmunity.* Dec;41 (8):601–10. PMID:18958762.

Favaro, A. 2009. *The Liberation Treatment: A Whole New Approach to MS.* Documentary. W5 CTV News aired November 21. Available online at http:// www.ctv.ca/servlet/ArticleNews/story/ CTVNews/20091120/W5_libera tion_091121/20091121?s_name=W5 (accessed November 22, 2009).

Favaro, A. 2010. *The Liberation War: Why MS Patients Aren't Waiting for Proof.* Documentary. W5 CTV News aired April 10. Available online at http://www.ctv.ca/servlet/ArticleNews/story/CTVNews/20100409/w5_liberation_update_100409/20100410?s_name=W5 (accessed June 13, 2010).

FDA 2010. Monograph for Mitoxantrone available at: http//:www.fda.gov (accessed 7/28/2010).

Ferlini, A., M. Bovolenta, M. Neri, F. Gualandi, A. Balboni, A. Yuryev, F. Salvi, D. Gemmati, A. Liboni, and P. Zamboni. 2010. "Custom CGH array profiling of copy number variations (CNVs) on chromosome 6p21.32 (HLA locus) in patients with venous malformations associated with multiple sclerosis." BMC Medical Genetics. 2010 Apr 28;11:64. PMID:20426824.

Filippi, M., M. Bozzali, M. Rovaris, O. Gonen, C. Kesavadas, A. Ghezzi, V. Martinelli, R. Grossman, G. Scotti, G. Comi, and A. Falani. 2003. "Evidence for widespread damage at the earliest stage of MS." *Brain.* Feb;126(Part 2):433–37. PMID:12538409.

Fischbach, F.A., D.W. Gregory, P.M. Harrison, T.G. Hoy, and J.M. Williams. 1971. "On the structure of hemosiderin and its relationship to ferritin." *Journal of Ultrastructure Research.* Dec;37(5): 495–503. PMID: 5136270.

Fisniku, L., P. Brex, D. Altman, K. Miszkiel, C. Benton, R. Lanyon, A. Thompson, and D. Miller. 2008. "Disability and T2 MRI lesions: a 20-year follow-up of patients with relapse onset of multiple sclerosis." *Brain.* Mar;131(Part 3):808–17. PMID:18234696.

Fog, T. 1965. "The topography of plaques in multiple sclerosis." *Acta Neurologica Scandinavica.* 1965;15:1–161. PMID:5213727.

Francesci, C. 2009. "The unsolved puzzle of multiple sclerosis and venous func-

tion." Comment in *The Journal of Neurosurgery and Psychiatry.* Apr;80:358. PMID:19289474.

Fraser, J., and T. Proft. 2007. "Superantigens and superallergens." *Chemical Immunology and Allergy.* 93:1–23. PMID: 17369697.

Friedman, T. 2005. *The World Is Flat: A Brief History of the Twenty-first Century.* New York: Farrar, Straus & Giroux.

Frohman, E., M. Racke, and C. Raine. 2006. "Multiple sclerosis — the plaque and its pathogensis." *New England Journal of Medicine.* Mar;354:942–55. PMID:16510748.

Ge, Y., V.M. Zohrabian, E.O. Osa, J. Xu, H. Jaggi, J. Herbert, E.M. Haacke, and R.I. Grossman. 2009. "Diminished visibility of cerebral venous vasculature in multiple sclerosis by susceptibility-weighted imaging at 3.0 Tesla." *Journal of Magnetic Resonance Imaging.* May;29 (5):1190–94. PMID:19388109.

Giles, J. 2006. "Drug trials: stacking the deck." *Nature.* Mar;440(16):270–72. Available online at http://www.nature.com/nature/journal/v440/n7082/full/440270a.html (accessed August 17, 2010).

Godley, M. 2010. CCSVI press conference at False Creek healthcare center. March 5, 2010. Available online at http://www.youtube.com/watch?v=8ocSlIfTxMs&feature=related (accessed July 10, 2010).

Grady, D. 2010. "From MS patients, outcry for unapproved treatment." *New York Times,* June 28, 2010.

Green, J. 2010. "Protesters rally for access to MS treatment." *Montreal Gazette,* May 6 2010.

Gutcher, I., and B. Becher. 2007. "APC-derived cytokines and t-cell polarization in autoimmune inflammation." *The Journal of Clinical Investigation.* May; 117(5):1119–17. PMID:17476341.

Gutiérrez, J., J. Linares-Palomino, C.

Lopez-Espada, M. Rodríguez, E. Ros, G. Piédrola, and M.C. del Maroto. 2001. "Chlamydia pneumoniae DNA in the arterial wall of patients with peripheral vascular disease." *Infection.* Aug;29(4):196–200. PMID:11545479.

Haacke, E.M. 2010a. *A brief history of the early venous vascular changes in MS.* Available online at http://www.ms-mri.com/history.php (accessed January 11, 2010).

Haacke, E.M. 2010b. *Proposal and protocol for testing using SWI MR I.* Available online at http://www.ms-mri.com (accessed March 20, 2010).

Haacke, E.M. 2010c. *Measuring iron, oxygen saturation and veins with SWI and SWIM: The clinical importance of vascular and hemodynamic information in studying neurodegenerative disease.* PowerPoint presentation given in Shanghai, April 10, 2010.

Haacke, E.M. 2010d. *MR Venography in CCSVI: the role of MRI in treatment.* PowerPoint presentation given in Detroit, August 2010. Available online at http://www.youtube.com/watch?v=1fQckdv3vAc (accessed August 31, 2010).

Haacke, E.M., J. Garbern, Y. Miao, C. Habib, and M. Liu. 2010. "Iron stores in cerebral veins in multiple sclerosis studied by susceptibility weighted imaging." *International Angiology.* Apr; 29(2):149–57. PMID:20351671.

Habib, C., W. Zheng, E.M. Haacke, S. Webb, and H. Nichol. 2010. "Visualizing iron deposition in multiple sclerosis cadaver brains." *6th International Conference on Medical Applications of Synchrotron Radiation* AIP Conference Proceedings, Volume 1266, 78–83.

Hafler, D., and A. Windhagen. 1995. *Neural Notes* 1(3):1–6.

Hammond, K., M. Metcalf, L. Carvajal, D. Okuda, R. Srinivasan, D. Vigneron, S. Nelson, D. Pelletier. 2008. "Quantitative in vivo magnetic resonance imaging of multiple sclerosis at 7 Tesla with sensitivity to iron." *Annals of Neurology.* Dec;64(6):707–13. PMID:19107998.

Heijmen, R.H., T.L. Bollen, D.A. Duyndam, T.T. Overtoom, J.C. Van Den Berg, and F.L. Moll. 2001. "Endovascular venous stenting in May-Thurner syndrome." *The Journal of Cardiovascular Surgery* (Torino). Feb;42(1):83–87. PMID:11292912.

Hemmer, B., J. Archelos, and H.P. Hartung. 2002. "New concepts in the pathogenesis of multiple sclerosis." *Nature Reviews Neuroscience.* Apr;3(4):291–301. PMID:11967559.

Henderson, A.P., M.H. Barnett, J.D. Parratt, and J.W. Prineas. 2009. Multiple sclerosis: distribution of inflammatory cells in newly forming lesions. *Annals of Neurology* Dec;66(6):739–53. PMID:20035511.

Hojnacki, D., P. Zamboni, A. Lopez-Soriano, R. Galleotti, E. Menegatti, B. Weinstock-Guttman, C. Schirda, C. Magnano, A.M. Malagoni, C. Kennedy, I. Bartolomei, F. Salvi, and R. Zivadinov. 2010. "Use of neck magnetic resonance venography, Doppler sonography and selective venography for diagnosis of chronic cerebrospinal venous insufficiency: a pilot study in multiple sclerosis patients and healthy controls." *International Angiology.* Apr; 29(2):127–39. PMID:20351669.

Hrobjartsson, A., and P. Gotzsche. 2010. "Placebo interventions for all clinical conditions." *Cochrane Database System Review.* Jan 20;(1):CD003974. PMID:20091554.

Hubbard, D. 2010. "The fMRI BOLD response in MS, support for the CCSVI hypothesis." Hubbard Foundation for fMRI Research (grant request).

James, T., M.A. Hughes, G.W. Cherry, and R.P. Taylor. 2003. "Evidence of oxidative stress in chronic venous ulcers." *Wound Repair and Regeneration.* May–Jun;11(3):172–76. PMID:12753 597.

Jonas, E., S. Schulz-Hardt, D. Frey, and N. Thelan. 2001. "Confirmation bias in sequential information search after preliminary decisions: an expansion of dissonance theoretical research on selective exposure to information." *Journal of Personality and Social Psychology.* Apr;80(4):557–71. PMID:11316221.

Jonez, H. 1952. "Management of multiple sclerosis." *Postgrad Med.* 1952;2:415–22.

Khan, O., F. Massimo, M. Freedman, F. Barkhof, P. Dore-Duffy, H. Lassmann, B. Trapp, A. Bar-Or, I. Zak, M. Siegal, and R. Lisak. 2010. "Chronic cerebrospinal venous insufficiency and multiple sclerosis." *Annals of Neurology.* Mar;67(3):286–90.

King, L., C. Stratton, and W. Mitchell. 2001. "Chlamydia pneumoniae in chronic skin wounds: a focused review." *The Journal of Investigative Dermatology Symposium Proceedings.* Dec;6(3):233–37. PMID:11924834.

Krasulova, E., M. Trneny, T. Kozal, B. Vackova, D. Pohlreich, D. Kemlink, P. Kobylka, I. Kovarova, P. Lhotakova, and E. Havrdova. 2010. "High-dose immunoablation with autologous haematopoietic stem cell transplantation in aggressive multiple sclerosis: a single centre 10-year experience." *Multiple Sclerosis.* Jun;16(6):685–93. PMID: 20350962.

Kremenchutzky, M., G. Rice, J. Baskerville, D. Wingerchuk, and G. Ebers. 2006. "The natural history of multiple sclerosis: a geographically based study 9: observations on the progressive phase of the disease." *Brain.* Mar;129(Part 3):584–94. PMID:16401620.

Krogias, C., A. Schroder, H. Wiendl, R. Hohfeld, and R. Gold. 2010. "'Chronic cerebrospinal venous insufficiency' and multiple sclerosis: a critical analysis and first observation in an unselected cohort of MS patients." *Der Nervenarzt.* Jun;81(6):740–46. PMID:20386873.

Kurtzke, J., and A. Heltberg. 2001. "Multiple sclerosis in the Faroe Islands an epitome." *The Journal of Clinical Epidemiology.* Jan;54(1):1–22. PMID:1116 5464.

Kurtzke, J., and K. Hyllestad. 1979. "Multiple sclerosis in the Faroe Islands: clinical and epidemiological features." *Annals of Neurology.* Jan;5(1):6–21. PMID:371519.

Kutzelnigg, A., C.F. Lucchinetti, C. Stadelmann, W. Brück, H. Rauschka, M. Bergmann, M. Schmidbauer, J.E. Parisi, and H. Lassmann. 2005. "Cortical demyelination and diffuse white matter injury in multiple sclerosis." *Brain.* Nov;128(Part 11):2705–12. PMID:16230320.

Kwidzinski, E., L.K. Mutlu, A.D. Kovac, J. Bunse, J. Goldmann, J. Mahlo, O. Aktas, F. Zipp, T. Kamradt, R. Nitsch, and I. Bechmann. 2003. "Self-tolerance in the immune privileged CNS: lessons from the entorhinal cortex lesion model." *Journal of Neural Transmission Supplementum.* 2003;(65):29–49. PMID:12946047.

Labropoulos, N., M. Borge, K. Pierce, and P. Pappas. 2007. "Criteria for defining significant central vein stenosis using duplex ultrasound." *Journal of Vascular Surgery.* Jul;46:101–7. PMID: 17540535.

Laino, C. 2010. "New theory on MS and CCSVI needs further study experts say." *Neurology Today.* June;10(12):28–29. DOI: 1097/01.NT.0000383489. 93815.43.

Laska, T., and K. Hannig. 2001. "Difficult therapy for spinal accessory nerve injury complicated by adhesive capsulitis." *Physical Therapy.* Mar;81(3):936–44. PMID:11268158.

Lassmann, H. 2003. "Hypoxia-like tissue injury as a component of multiple sclerosis lesions." *Journal of the Neurological Sciences*. Feb 15;206(2):187–91. PMID: 12559509.

Lavi, E., and C. Constantinescu (eds). 2005. *Experimental Models of Multiple Sclerosis*. New York: Springer Science & Business Media.

Law, M., A.M. Saindane, Y. Ge, J.S. Babb, G. Johnson, L.J. Mannon, J. Herbert, and R.I. Grossman. 2004. "Microvascular abnormality in relapsing remitting multiple sclerosis: perfusion MR imaging findings in normal appearing white matter." *Radiology*. Jun;231(3):645–52. PMID:15163806.

Lee, B., J. Bergen, P. Gloviczki, J. Laredo, D. Loose, R. Mattassi, K. Parsi, J. Villavicencio, and P. Zamboni. 2009. "Diagnosis and treatment of venous malformations consensus document of the International Union of Phlebology (IUP) 2009." *International Angiology*. Dec;28(6):434–51. PMID:20087280.

Lee, B., J. Laredo, and R. Neville. 2010. "Embryological background of truncular venous malformation in the extracranial venous pathways as the cause of chronic cerebro spinal venous insufficiency." *International Angiology*. Apr;29(2):95–108. PMID:20351665.

Lensing, A., H. Buller, P. Pradoni, D. Batchelor, A. Molenaar, A. Cogo, M. Vigo, P. Huismen, and J. ten Cate. 1992. "Contrast venography, the gold standard for the diagnosis of deep vein thrombosis: improvement in observer agreement." *Journal of Thrombosis and Haemostasis*. Jan 23;67(1):8–12 PMID:1615489.

Leon, M. 1998. Interview with unlisted author for Angioplasty.org. Transcript available at http://www.ptca.org/nv/in terviews.html (accessed August 21, 2010).

LeVine, S. 1997. "Iron deposits in multiple sclerosis and Alzheimer's disease brains." *Brain Research*. Jun 20;760(1–2):298–303. PMID:9237552.

Levy, E., and E. Lang. 2010. "Liberation or Placebo Effect?" *Montreal Gazette*, August 24, 2010.

Lipton, H., A. Kumar, and M. Trottier. 2005. "Theiler's virus persistence in the central nervous system of mice is associated with continuous viral replication and the difference in outcome of infection of infiltrating macrophages versus oligodendrocytes." *Virus Research*. Aug; 111(2):214–23. PMID:15893838.

Lo, B. 2010. "Serving two masters — conflicts of interest in academic medicine." *New England Journal of Medicine*. Feb 25;362(8):669–71. PMID:20181 969.

Lucchinetti, C., W. Brück, J. Parisi, B. Scheithauer, M. Rodriguez, and H. Lassmann. 2000. "Heterogeneity of multiple sclerosis lesions: implications for the pathogenesis of demyelination." *Annals of Neurology*. Jun;47(6):707–17. PMID:10852536.

MacDonald, S. 2010. Testimony on June 6, 2010, for the Canadian Parliament regarding CCSVI. Available online at http://www.youtube.com/user/famille joyeuse#p/u/6/KVfmCJLUyIc (accessed June 14, 2010).

Malagoni, A., R. Galeotti, E. Menegatti, F. Manfredini, N. Basaglia, F. Salvi, and P. Zamboni. 2010. " Is chronic fatigue the symptom of venous insufficiency associated with multiple sclerosis? A longitudinal pilot study." *International Angiology*. Apr;29:176–82. PMID:20351673.

Markowitz, C. 2007. "Interferon beta mechanism of action and dosing issues." *Neurology*. Jun 12;68(24 Suppl 4):S8–11. PMID:17562848.

Marrie, R.A., R. Rudick, R. Horwitz, G. Cutter, T. Tyry, D. Campagnolo, and T. Vollmer. 2010. "Vascular comorbidity is associated with more rapid disability progression in multiple sclerosis." *Neurology.* Mar 30;74(13):1041–47. PMID:20350978.

Martinelli, V., M. Radaelli, L. Straffi, M. Rodegher, and G. Comi. 2009. "Mitoxantrone: benefits and risks in multiple sclerosis patients." *Neurological Sciences.* Oct;30 Suppl 2:S167–70. PMID:19882368.

McAlpine, D., and A. Compston. 2006. *McAlpine's Multiple Sclerosis.* Philadelphia: Churchill Livingstone Elesevier.

McDonald, I., A. Compston, G. Edan, D. Goodkin, H. Hartung, F. Lublin, H. McFarland, D. Paty, C. Polman, S. Reingold, M. Sandberg-Wollheim, W. Sibley, A. Thompson, S. van den Noort, B. Weinshenker, and J. Wolinsky. 2001. "Recommended diagnostic criteria for multiple sclerosis: guidelines from the international panel on the diagnosis of multiple sclerosis." *Annals of Neurology.* Jul;50:121–27. PMID:11456302.

McTigue, D., and R. Tripathi. 2008. "The life, death, and replacement of oligodendrocytes in the adult CNS." *The Journal of Neurochemistry.* Oct;107 (1):1–19. PMID:18643793.

Menegatti, E., V. Genova, M. Tessari, A.M. Malagoni, I. Bartolomei, M. Zuolo, R. Galeotti, F. Salvi, and P. Zamboni. 2010. "The reproducibility of colour Doppler in chronic cerebrospinal venous insufficiency associated with multiple sclerosis." *International Angiology.* Apr;29(2):121–26. PMID:20351668.

Menegatti, E., and P. Zamboni. 2008. "Doppler haemodynamics of cerebral venous return." *Current Neurovascular Research.* Nov;5(4):260–65. Review. PMID:18991660.

Metz, I., C. Lucchinetti, H. Openshaw, A. Garcia-Merino, H. Lassmann, M. Freedman, H. Atkins, B. Azzarelli, O.

Kolar, and W. Bruck. 2007. "Autologous haematopoietic stem cell transplantation fails to stop demyelination and neurodegeneration in multiple sclerosis." *Brain.* May;130(Part 5): 1254–62. PMID:17293360.

Michiels, C., N. Bouaziz, and J. Remacle. 2002. "Hypoxia-induced activation of endothelial cells as a possible cause of venous diseases: hypothesis." *International Angiology.* Jun;21(2 Suppl 1):18–25. PMID:12515976.

Miller, D., F. Barkhof, J. Frank, G. Parker, and J. Thompson. 2002. "Measurement of brain atrophy in multiple sclerosis: pathological basis, methodological aspects and clinical relevance." *Brain* Aug;125(8):1676–95. PMID:12135961.

Mitsuhashi, T., R. Morris, and H. Ives. 1991. "1,25-dihydroxyvitamin D3 modulates growth of vascular smooth muscle cells." *The Journal of Clinical Investigation.* Jun;87(6):1889–95. PMID:1645744.

Modin, H., W. Olsson, J. Hillert, and T. Masterman. 2004. "Modes of action of HLA-DR susceptibility specificities in multiple sclerosis." *American Journal of Human Genetics.* June;74(6):1321–22. PMID:15195659.

Munger, K., S. Zhang, and E. O'Reilly. 2004. "Vitamin D intake and incidence of multiple sclerosis." *Neurology.* Jan 13;62(1):60–65. PMID:14718698.

Muraro, P., R. Cassiani Igoni, and R. Martin. 2003. "Hematopoeitic stem cell transplantation for multiple sclerosis: current status and future challenges." *Current Opinion in Neurology.* Jun;16(3):299–305. PMID:12858065.

Murray, T.J. 2005. *Multiple Sclerosis: The History of the Disease.* New York: Demos Medical Publishing.

Murrell, T.G., L.S. Harbige, and I.C. Robinson. 1991. "A review of the aetiology of multiple sclerosis: an ecological approach." *Annals of Human Biology.* Mar–Apr;18(2):95–112. PMID:2024 951.

Nash, R., O. Stuve, J. Bowen, E. Frohman, L. Griffith, G. Hutton, G. Kraft, U. Popat, M. Racke, and P. Murano. 2008. "Autologous HSCT for advanced MS: glass half empty or half full?" *Brain.* Feb;131(Part 2):e89. PMID:17908695.

Neema, M., A. Arora, B.C. Healy, Z.D. Guss, S.D. Brass, Y. Duan, G.J. Buckle, B.I. Glanz, L. Stazzone, S.J. Khoury, H.L. Weiner, C.R. Guttmann, and R. Bakshi. 2009. *Journal of Neuroimaging.* Jan;19(1):3–8. PMID:19192042.

Nicolson, M., and C. McLaughlin. 1987. "Social constructionism and medical sociology: a study of the vascular theory of MS" *Society of Health Illness.* Available online at http://onlinelibrary.wiley.com/doi/10.1111/1467-9566.ep1134 0153/pdf (accessed August 17, 2010).

Njenga, M., K. Pavelco, J. Baisch, X. Lin, C. David, J. Leibowitz, and M. Rodriguez. 1996. "Theiler's virus persistence and demyelination in MHC deficient mice." *Journal of Virology.* Mar; 70(3):1729–37. PMID:8627694.

NMSS (National Multiple Sclerosis Society). 2010. Grant Awards. http://www.nationalmssociety.org (accessed June 14, 2010).

Nos, C., J. Sastre-Garriga, C. Borras, J. Rio, M. Tintore, and X. Montalban. 2004. "Clinical impact of intravenous methylprednisolone in attacks of multiple sclerosis." *Multiple Sclerosis.* Aug; 10(4):413–16. PMID:15327039.

Opexa. 2008. "Opexa announces top-line results from phase IIb clinical trial of Tovaxin for the treatment of multiple sclerosis." Available online at http://businesswire.com/portal/site/opexa/ (accessed June 10, 2009).

Opsahl, M., and P. Kennedy. 2005. "Early and late HHV6 gene transcripts in multiple sclerosis lesions and normal appearing white matter." *Brain.* Mar;128(Part 3):516–27. PMID:1565 9422.

Ormiston, J.A., P.W. Serruys, E. Regar, D. Dudek, L. Thuesen, M.W. Webster, Y. Onuma, H.M. Garcia-Garcia, R. McGreevy, and S. Veldhof. 2008. "A bioabsorbable everolimus-eluting coronary stent system for patients with single de-novo coronary artery lesions (ABSORB): a prospective open-label trial." *Lancet.* Mar 15;371(9616):899–907. PMID:18342684.

O'Shea, C. 2010. "Heart superdoc calls foot dragging on CCSVI 'unethical.'" *Online Journal.* Available online at http://for-greet.squarespace.com/journal/tag/gianfranco-camplani.

Pert, C. 2000. *Your Body Is Your Subconscious Mind.* Lecture on CD. Louisville, CO: Sounds True Publishing.

Petito, C., J. Olarte, B. Roberts, T. Nowak, and W. Pulsinelli. 1998. "Selective glial vulnerability in transient global ischemia in rat brain." *The Journal of Neuropathology and Experimental Neurology.* Mar;57(3):231–38. PMID:960 0215.

Philips, L. 2010. "This way in: CCSVI and multiple sclerosis." *Neurology Now.* Jul/Aug;6(4):9–11. DOI:10.1097/01.NN N.0000387765.20876.4c.

Pirko, I., and R. Zivadinov. 2009. "Transcranial sonography of deep gray nuclei: a new outcome measure in multiple sclerosis?" *Neurology.* Sep;73:1006–7. PMID:19710403.

Pittock, S., R. McLelland, W. Mayr, N. Jorgensen, B. Weinshenker, and M. Rodriguiz. 2004. "Clinical implications of benign MS a 20-year population-based follow-up study." *Annals of Neurology.* Aug;56(2): 303–6. PMID:15293286.

Pittock, S., B. Weinshenker, J. Noseworthy, C. Lucchinetti, M. Keegan, D. Wingerchuk, J. Carter, E. Shuster, and

M. Rodriguiz. 2006. "Not every patient with multiple sclerosis should be treated at time of diagnosis." Comment in *Archives of Neurology*. Apr;63 (4):611–12. PMID:16606780.

Plasmati, R., F. Pastorelli, N. Fini, F. Salvi, R. Galeotti, and P. Zamboni. 2010. "Chronic cerebro-spinal venous insufficiency: report of transcranial magnetic stimulation follow-up study in a patient with multiple sclerosis." *International Angiology*. Apr;29(2):189–92. PMID:20351675.

Pohl, D., K. Rostasy, C. Jacobi, P. Lange, R. Nau, B. Krone, and F. Hanefeld. 2010. "Intrathecal antibody production against Epstein-Barr and other neurotropic viruses in pediatric and adult onset multiple sclerosis." *The Journal of Neurology*. Feb;257(2):212–16. PM ID:19714396.

Prineas, J. 1985. "The neuropathology of multiple sclerosis." In *The Handbook of Clinical Neurology*, ed. J.C. Koetsier (rev. ed). Vol. 3(47):213–57. New York: Elesevier.

Prineas, J. 1994. "The pathology of multiple sclerosis." In *Multiple Sclerosis: Current Status of Research and Treatment*, eds. R. Herndon and F. Seil. New York: Demos, 113–30.

Prineas, J. 2009. Interview by the Australian NMSS following the Charcot Award. Available online at http://www. msif.org/en/research/msif_research_aw ards/2009_charcot.html (accessed April 23, 2010).

Putnam, T. 1935. "Encephalitis and sclerotic plaques produced by venular obstruction." *Archives of Neurology and Psychiatry*. 1935;33(5):929–40.

Putnam, T. 1937. "Evidences of vascular occlusion and encephalomyelitis." *Archives of Neurology and Psychiatry*. 1937;37(6):1298–1321.

Qui, W., S. Raven, J.S. Wu, W.M. Carroll, F.L. Mastaglia, and A.G. Ker-

mode. 2010. "Wedge shaped medullary lesions in MS." *Journal of the Neurological Sciences*. Mar 15;290(1–2):190–93. PMID:20056253.

Quintana, C. 2007. "About the presence of hemosiderin in the hippocampus of Alzheimers patients." *The Journal of Alzheimers Disease*. Sept;12(2):157–60. PMID:17917160.

Raferty, J. 2010. "Multiple sclerosis risk sharing scheme: a costly failure." *British Medical Journal*. 2010;340:c16 72. Available online at http://www. bmj.com/cgi/content/extract/340/jun0 3_1/c1672 (accessed August 17, 2010).

Raffetto, J., and R. Khalil. 2008. "Matrix metalloproteinases in venous tissue remodeling and varicose vein formation." *Current Vascular Pharmacology*. Jul;6(3): 158–72. PMID:18673156.

Raine, C. 2008. "Multiple sclerosis: classification revisited reveals homogeneity and recapitulation." *Annals of Neurology*. Jan;63(1):1–3. PMID:18232014.

Rice, G., M. Filippi, and G. Comi. 2000. "Cladribine and progressive MS: clinical and MRI outcomes of a multicenter controlled trial Cladribine MRI Study Group." *Neurology*. Mar 14;54(5):1145–55. PMID:10720289.

Rindfleisch, E. 1863. "Histologisches detail zu der grauen degeneration von gehirn und ruckenmark." *Archives of Pathological Anatomy and Physiology*. 1863;26:474–83.

Roach, E. 2004. "Is multiple sclerosis an autoimmune disorder?" *Archives of Neurology*. Oct;61(10):1615–16. PMID: 15477522.

Rock, R.B., G. Gekker, S. Hu, W. Sheng, M. Cheeran, J. Lokensgard, and P. Peterson. 2004. "Role of microglia in central nervous system infections." *Clinical Microbiology Reviews*. Oct; 17(4):942–64. PMID:15489356.

Rogojan, C., and J. Frederiksen. 2009. "Hematopoietic stem cell transplantation in multiple sclerosis." *Acta Neuro-logica Scandinavica.* Dec;120(6):371–82. PMID:19785643.

Rolak, L. 2009. "The history of MS." NMSS brochure. Available online at http://www.nationalmultiplesclerosis society.org (accessed January 22, 2010).

Roubin, G. 2005. Interview for Angio-plasty.org video library. Available online at http://www.pcta.org (accessed August 10, 2010).

Saccardi, R., et al. (42 authors). 2006. "Autologous stem cell transplantation for progressive multiple sclerosis: up-date of the European Group for Blood and Marrow Transplantation autoim-mune diseases working party database." *Multiple Sclerosis.* Dec;12(6):814–23. PMID:17263012.

Salvi, F. 2010. Interview with CCSVI Al-liance, July 26, 2010. Available online at http://www.ccsvialliance.org. (ac-cessed August 27, 2010).

Samson, K. 2010. "Experimental multiple sclerosis vascular shunting procedure halted at Stanford." *Annals of Neurol-ogy.* Jan;67(1):a13–15. PMID:201868 48.

Scalfari, A., A. Neuhaus, A. Degenhardt, G. Rice, P. Muraro, M. Daumer, and G. Ebers. 2010. "The natural history of multiple sclerosis: a geographically based study 10: relapses and long term disability." *Brain.* Jul;133(Part 7):584–94. PMID:20534650.

Schelling, A.F. 2004. "Multiple sclerosis: the image and its message. The mean-ing of the classic lesion forms." Avail-able online at http://www.ms-info.net (accessed December 20, 2008).

Scholz, D., et al. 2000. "Ultrastructure and molecular histology of rabbit hind-limb collateral artery growth (arterio-genesis)." *Virchows Archive.* Mar;436 (3):257–70. PMID:10782885.

Schwartz, M., and J. Kipnis. 2002. "Mul-tiple sclerosis as a by-product of the failure to maintain protective autoim-munity." *The Neuroscientist.* Oct;8(5): 405–13. PMID:12374425.

Schwid, S., and R. Gross. 2005. "Bias, not conflict of interest, is the enemy." *Neurology* (editorial). 2005;64:1830–31.

Simka, M. 2008. "How to skip the 'false, trivial, obvious' paradigm." *Medical Hypotheses.* Nov;71(5):817. PMID:186 91829.

Simka, M. 2009a. "Refluxing blood in the cerebral and spinal veins a potential agent of the initiation of multiple scle-rosis." *Phlebology Review.* 17(1):51–56. Available online at http://www.insight-library.net/?nodeid=journals&_ap_righ t_content_stage=show_article&_ap_rig ht_content_article_id=1213# (volume 17, issue 1).

Simka, M. 2009b. "Biophysics of venous return from the brain from the perspec-tive of pathophysiology of multiple sclerosis." Unpublished work, private collection.

Simka, M. 2009c. "Blood brain barrier compromise with endothelial inflam-mation may lead to autoimmune loss of myelin during multiple sclerosis." *Current Neurovascular Research.* May; 6(2):132–39. PMID:9442163.

Simka, M. 2009d. "Chronic cerebrospinal venous insufficiency: a potential weak-ening factor in the blood brain barrier." *The Journal of Neurology, Neurosurgery and Psychiatry.* Comment on "Chronic cerebrospinal venous insufficiency," by Zamboni et al., Apr;80(4):392–99. PMID:19060024.

Simka, M. 2010a. "Reinterpreting the MR signs of hemodynamic impairment in the brains of multiple sclerosis pa-tients from the perspective of a recent discovery of outflow block in extracra-nial veins." *The Journal of Neuroscience Research.* Feb 1 (epub ahead of print). PMID:20127806.

Simka, M. 2010b. "Cellular and molecular mechanisms of venous leg ulcers development the 'puzzle' theory." *International Angiology*. Feb;29(1):1–19.

Simka, M. 2010c. Letter to the Canadian Parliamentary Subcommittee on Neurological Diseases. Available online at http://www.facebook.com/notes/ms-ccsvi-uk/dr-simkas-letter-to-the-canadian-parliament/10150257759150713 (accessed September 1, 2010).

Simka, M., J. Kostecki, M. Zaniewski, E. Majewski, and D. Szewczyk-Urgacz. 2009. "Preliminary report on pathologic flow patterns in the internal jugular and vertebral veins of patients with multiple sclerosis." *Phlebology Review*. 17(2):61–64. Available online at http://www.insight-library.net/?nodeid=journals&_ap_right_content_stage=show_article&_ap_right_content_article_id=1213# (accessed August 18, 2010).

Simka, M., J. Kostecki, M. Zaniewski, E. Majewski, and M. Hartel. 2010a. "Extracranial Doppler sonographic criteria of chronic cerebrospinal venous insufficiency in the patients with multiple sclerosis." *International Angiology*. Apr; 29(2):109–14. PMID:20351666.

Simka, M., T. Ludyga, M. Kazibudzki, A. Adamczyk-Ludyga, J. Wróbel, P. Latacz, J. Piegza, and M. Świerad. 2010b. "Correlation of localization and severity of extracranial venous lesions with clinical status of multiple sclerosis." Presented at ECTRIMS.

Simka, M., T. Ludyga, M. Kazibudzki, M. Hartel, M. Świerad, J. Piegza, P. Latacz, and L. Sedlak. 2010c. "Endovascular treatment for chronic cerebrospinal venous insufficiency: is the procedure safe?" In press.

Simka, M., and Z. Rybak. 2008. "Hypothetical molecular mechanisms by which local iron overload facilitates the development of venous leg ulcers and multiple sclerosis lesions." *Medical Hypotheses*. Aug;71(2):293–97. PMID: 18400414.

Singh, A.V., and P. Zamboni. 2009. "Anomalous venous blood flow and iron deposition in multiple sclerosis." *Journal of Cerebral Blood Flow and Metabolism*. Dec;29(12):1867–78. PMID: 19724286.

SIR (Society of Interventional Radiology). 2010. Position statement of the Society of Interventional Radiology concerning CCSVI. Available online at http://www.sirweb.org/news/newsPDF/Release_JVIR_MS_final.pdf.

Slonim, S., M. Dake, M. Razavi, S. Kee, S. Samuels, J. Rhee, and C. Semba. 1999. "Management of misplaced endovascular stents." *Journal of Vascular and Intervenional Radiology*. Jul–Aug; 10(7):851–59. PMID:10435701.

Somers, E., S. Thomas, L. Smeeth, and A. Hall. 2009. "Are individuals with an autoimmune disease at higher risk of a second autoimmune disorder?" *American Journal of Epidemiology*. Mar 15;169(6):749–55. PMID:19224981.

Srinivasan, R., N. Sailasuta, R. Hurd, S. Nelson, and D. Pelletier. 2005. "Evidence of elevated glutamate in multiple sclerosis using magnetic resonance spectroscopy at 3T." *Brain*. May;128 (Part 5):1016–25. PMID:15758036.

Sriram, S., and I. Steiner. 2005. "Experimental allergic encephalomyelitis: a misleading model of MS." *Annals of Neurology*. Dec;58(6):939–45. PMID: 16315280.

Stanbrook, M., and P. Hebert. 2010. "Access to treatment for multiple sclerosis must be based on science not hope." *Canadian Medical Association Journal*. DOI:10.1503/cmaj.100835.

Steinman, L., and S. Zamvil. 2005. "The virtues and pitfalls of EAE for the development of therapies for multiple sclerosis." *Trends in Immunology*. Nov; 26(11):565–71. PMID:16153891.

Stinissen, P., and N. Hellings. 2008. "Activation of myelin reactive T cells in multiple sclerosis: a possible role for T cell degeneracy?" *European Journal of Immunology.* May;38(5):1190–93. PMID:18435726.

Stoeckel, D., A. Pelton, and T. Duerig. 2004. "Self-expanding nitinol stents: material and design considerations." *European Radiology.* Feb;14(2):292–301. PMID:12955452.

Stratton, C., and D. Wheldon. 2007. "Antimicrobial treatment of multiple sclerosis." *Infection.* Oct;35(5):383–86. PMID:17882356.

Sugden, J., J. Davies, M. Witham, A. Morris, and A. Struthers. 2008. "Vitamin D improves endothelial function in patients with diabetes mellitus." *Diabetic Medicine.* Mar;25(3):320–25. PMID:18279409.

Sundstrom, P., A. Wahlin, K. Ambarki, R. Birgander, A. Eklund, and J. Malm. 2010. "Venous and cerebrospinal fluid flow in multiple sclerosis: a case control study." *Annals of Neurology.* Aug;68(2): 255–59. PMID:20695018.

Swiderski, R. 1998. *Multiple Sclerosis through History and Human Life.* Jefferson, NC: McFarland.

Symposium 2010. Symposium on CCSVI in Brooklyn, July 26, 2010. Multiple presentations. Physician speakers as noted in text. Videos available online at http://www.youtube.com/watch?v=tfweIvjWYuo (accessed August 31, 2010).

Talbert, D. 2008. "Raised venous pressure as a factor in multiple sclerosis." *Medical Hypotheses.* 2008;70(6):1112–17. PMID:18079069.

Tan, I., R. van Schijndel, P. Pouwels, M. van Walderveen, J. Reichenbach, R. Manoliu, and F. Barkhof. 2000. "MR venography of multiple sclerosis." *American Journal of Neuroradiology.* Jun–Jul;21(6):1039–42. PMID:10871010.

Trapani, J. 1995. "Target cell apoptosis induced by cytotoxic T cells and natural killer cells involves synergy between pore-forming protein, perforin and serine protease granzyme B." *Australian and New Zealand Journal of Medicine.* Dec;25(6):793–99. PMID:8770355.

Tremlett, H., D, Paty, and V. Devonshire. 2006. "Disability progression is slower in multiple sclerosis then previously reported." *Neurology.* Jan 24;66(2):172–77. PMID:16434648.

Tsai, J., and D. Gilden. 2001. "Chlamydia pneumoniae and multiple sclerosis: no significant association." *Trends in Microbiology.* Apr;9(4):152–54. PMID:11286864.

Tsutsui, S., and P. Stys. 2009. "Degeneration versus autoimmunity in MS." Comment in *Annals of Neurology.* Dec;66(6):712. PMID:20033985.

Turner, J., R. Deyo, J. Loeser, M. Von Korff, and W. Fordyce. 1994. "The importance of placebo effects in pain treatment and research." *Journal of the American Medical Association.* May 25;271(70):1609–14. PMID:7880221.

Ulkur, E., F. Yuksel, C. Acikel, and B. Celikoz. 2002. "Effect of hyperbaric oxygen on pedicle flaps with compromised circulation." *Microsurgery.* 2002; 22(1):16–20. PMID:11891870.

Vafiadaki, E., A. Reis, S. Keers, R. Harrison, L.V. Anderson, T. Raffelsberger, S. Ivanova, H. Hoger, R.E. Bittner, K. Bushby, and R. Bashir. 2001. "Cloning of the mouse dysferlin gene and genomic characterization of the SJL-Dysf mutation." *Neuroreport.* Mar 5;12(3): 625–29. PMID:11234777.

van Beek, J., K. Elward, and P. Gasque. 2003. "Activation of complement in the central nervous system: roles in neurodegeneration and protection." *Annals of the New York Academy of Sciences.* May;992:56–71. PMID:12794047.

Vandenbroucke, J. 2008. "Observational research, randomized trials, and two views of medical science." *Public Library of Science*. Mar 11;5(3):e67. PMID:18336067.

Visser, L., R. Beekman, C. Tijssen, B. Uitdehaag, M. Lee, K. Movig, and A. Lenderink. 2004. "A randomized, double-blind, placebo-controlled pilot study of i.v. immune globulins in combination with i.v. methylprednisolone in the treatment of relapses in patients with MS." *Multiple Sclerosis*. Feb;10 (1):89–91. PMID:14760960.

Vladmirova, O., J. O'Conner, A. Cahill, H. Alder, C. Butunoi, and B. Kalman. 1998. "Oxidative damage to DNA in plaques of MS brains." *Multiple Sclerosis*. Oct;4(5):413–18. PMID:9839301.

Walter, U., S. Wagner, S. Horowski, R. Benecke, and U.K. Zettl. 2009. "Transcranial brain sonography findings predict disease progression in multiple sclerosis." *Neurology*. Sep 29;73(13):1010–17. PMID:19657105.

Waubant, E., D. Goodkin, L. Gee, P. Bacchetti, R. Sloan, T. Stewart, P. Andersson, G. Stabler, and K. Miller. 1999. "Serum MMP-9 and TIMP-1 levels are related to MRI activity in relapsing multiple sclerosis." *Neurology*. Oct 22;53(7):1397–1401. PMID:10534241.

Wautier, J., C. Zoucourian, O. Chappey, M. Wautier, P. Guillausseau, R. Cao, O. Hori, D. Stern, and A. Schmidt. 1996. "Receptor mediated endothelial cell dysfunction in diabetic vasculopathy: soluble receptor for advanced glycation end products blocks hyperpermeability in rats." *The Journal of Clinical Investigation*. Jan;97(1):238–43. PMID:8550841.

Werring, D., D. Brassat, A.G. Droogan, C.A. Clark, M.R. Symms, G.J. Barker, D.G. MacManus, A.J. Thompson, and D.H. Miller. 2000. "The pathogenesis of lesions and normal-appearing white matter changes in multiple sclerosis: a serial diffusion MRI study." *Brain*. Aug;123 (Part 8):1667–76. PMID:10908196.

Wuerfel, J., J. Bellmann-Strobl, P. Brunecker, O. Aktas, H. McFarland, A. Villringer, and F. Zipp. 2004. "Changes in cerebral perfusion precede plaque formation in multiple sclerosis: a longitudinal perfusion MRI study." *Brain*. Jan;127(Part 1):111–19. PMID:14570816.

Xiayan, S., M. Tanaka, S. Kondo, K. Okamoto, and S. Hirai. 1998. "Clinical significance of reduced cerebral metabolism in multiple sclerosis: a combined PET and MRI study." *Annals of Nuclear Medicine*. Apr;12(2):89–94. PMID:9637279.

Yoles, E., E. Hauben, O. Palgi, E. Agranov, A. Gothilf, A. Cohen, V. Kuchroo, I.R. Cohen, H. Weiner, and M. Schwartz. 2001. "Protective autoimmunity is a physiological response to CNS trauma." *The Journal of Neuroscience*. Jun 1;21(11):3740–48. Erratum in *The Journal of Neuroscience* 2001 Aug 1; 21(15):1a. PMID:11356861.

Yao, S., P. Pandey, A. Ljunggren-Rose, and S. Sriram. 2010. "LPS mediated injury to oligodendrocytes is mediated by the activation of nNOS: relevance to human demyelinating disease." *Nitric Oxide*. Apr 1;22(3):197–204. PMID: 20005301.

Yevzlin, A., and A. Asif. 2009. "Stent placement in hemodialysis access: historical lessons, the state-of-the-art and future directions." *Clinical Journal of the American Society of Nephrology*. May;4(5):996–1008. Review. PMID: 19406965.

Zamboni, P. 2006. "The big idea: iron-dependent inflammation in venous disease and proposed parallels in MS."

Journal of the Royal Society of Medicine. Nov;99(11):589–93. PMID:17082306.

Zamboni, P. 2010. "Chronic cerebrospinal venous insufficiency." Editorial. *International Angiology.* Apr;29(2):91–92. PMID:20361663.

Zamboni, P., E. Menegatti, I. Bartolomei, R. Galeotti, A.M. Malagoni, G. Tacconi, and F. Salvi. 2007. "Intracranial venous haemodynamics in multiple sclerosis." *Current Neurovascular Research.* Nov;4(4):252–58. PMID:1804 5150.

Zamboni, P., A. Cossu, L. Carpanese, G. Simonetti, G. Masarelli, and A. Liboni. 1990. "The so called primary venous aneurysms." *Phlebology.* 1990;5:45–50.

Zamboni, P., S. Lanzara, F. Mascoli, A. Caggiati, A. Liboni. 2008. "Inflammation in venous disease." *International Angiology.* Oct;27(5):361–69. Review. PMID:18974697.

Zamboni, P., G. Consorti, R. Galeotti, S. Gianesini, E. Menegatti, G. Tacconi, and F. Carinci. 2009a. "Venous collateral circulation of the extracranial cerebrospinal outflow routes." *Current Neurovascular Research.* Aug;6(3):204–12. PMID:19534716.

Zamboni, P., R. Galeotti, E. Menegatti, A.M. Malagoni, S. Gianesini, I. Bartolomei, F. Mascoli, and F. Salvi. 2009b. "A prospective open-label study of endovascular treatment of chronic cerebrospinal venous insufficiency." *Journal of Vascular Surgery.* Dec;50(6):1348–58.e1–3. PMID:19958985.

Zamboni, P., R. Galeotti, E. Menegatti, A.M. Malagoni, G. Tacconi, S. Dall'Ara, I. Bartolomei, and F. Salvi. 2009c. "Chronic cerebrospinal venous insufficiency in patients with multiple sclerosis." *The Journal of Neurosurgery and Psychiatry.* Apr;80(4):392–99. PMID:19060024.

Zamboni, P., E. Menegatti, R. Galeotti, A.M. Malagoni, G. Tacconi, S. Dall'Ara, I. Bartolomei, and F. Salvi. 2009d. "The value of cerebral Doppler venous haemodynamics in the assessment of multiple sclerosis." *Journal of Neurological Sciences.* Jul 15;282(1–2):21–27. PMID:19144359.

Zamboni, P., E. Menegatti, B. Weinstock-Guttman, C. Schirda, J.L. Cox, A.M. Malagoni, D. Hojanacki, C. Kennedy, E. Carl, M.G. Dwyer, N. Bergsland, R. Galeotti, S. Hussein, I. Bartolomei, F. Salvi, and R. Zivadinov. 2009e. "The severity of chronic cerebrospinal venous insufficiency in patients with multiple sclerosis is related to altered cerebrospinal fluid dynamics." *Functional Neurology.* Jul–Sep;24(3):133–38. PMID:20018140.

Zamboni, P., E. Menegatti, B. Weinstock-Guttman, C. Schirda, J.L. Cox, A. Malagoni, D. Hojnacki, C. Kennedy, E. Carl, M. Dwyer, N. Bergsland, R. Galleotti, S. Hussein, I. Bartolomei, F. Salvi, M. Ramanathan, and R. Zivadinov. 2010. "CSF dynamics and brain volume in multiple sclerosis are associated with extracranial venous flow anomalies: a pilot study." *International Angiology.* Apr;29(2):140–48. PMID:20351637.

Zhang, L., B. Zhang, J. Zhang, and H. Zhang. 2007. "Immune function of erythrocytes in patients with chronic venous insufficiency of the lower extremity." *Chinese Medical Journal* (English). Dec 20;120(24):2224–28. PMID:18167207.

Zhang, Y., R. Zabad, X. Wei, L. Metz, M. Hill, and J. Mitchell. 2007. "Deep grey matter 'black T2' on 3 Tesla magnetic resonance imaging correlates with disability in multiple sclerosis." *Multiple Sclerosis.* Aug;13(7):880–83. PMID:17 468444.

Zivadinov, R. 2010. Transcript of live Web forum proctored by the AAN and NMSS: CCSVI and what it could mean to people living with multiple sclerosis. Includes discussion of early CTEVD results. Broadcast live from Toronto, Canada, April 14, 2010.

Zivadinov, R., C. Schirda, M.G. Dwyer, M.E. Haacke, B. Weinstock-Guttman, E. Menegatti, M. Heininen-Brown, C. Magnano, A.M. Malagoni, D.S. Wack, D. Hojnacki, C. Kennedy, E. Carl, N. Bergsland, S. Hussein, G. Poloni, I. Bartolomei, F. Salvi, and P. Zamboni. 2010. "Chronic cerebrospinal venous insufficiency and iron deposition on susceptibility-weighted imaging in patients with multiple sclerosis: a pilot case-control study." *International Angiology*. Apr;29(2):158–75. PMID:203 51672.

Index

Page numbers in ***bold italics*** indicate illustrations.